GETTING RESEARCH FINDINGS
INTO PRACTICE

Second edition

GETTING RESEARCH FINDINGS INTO PRACTICE

Second edition

Edited by Andrew Haines and Anna Donald

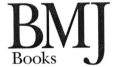

First published in 1998
Second impression 2000
Second edition 2002
by BMJ Books, BMA House, Tavistock Square,
London WC1H 9JR

www.bmjbooks.com

British Library Cataloguing in Publication Data

A catalogue record for this book is available from the
British Library

ISBN 0-7279-1553-3

Typeset by Newgen Imaging Systems (P) Ltd., Chennai, India
Printed and bound in Spain by GraphyCems, Navarra

Contents

Contributors

David Armstrong, Reader in Medical Sociology, Department of General Practice, King's College, London, UK

Ione Auston, Librarian, National Information Center on Health Services Research and HealthCare Technology (NICHSR), National Library of Medicine, Washington DC, USA

Lisa Bero, Professor, Institute for Health Policy Studies and Department of Clinical Pharmacy, University of California, San Francisco, USA

David Braunholtz, Senior Research Fellow, Department of Public Health and Epidemiology, University of Birmingham, Birmingham, UK

Jiri Chard, Research and Development Project Officer, Department of Public Health and Epidemiology, University of Birmingham, Birmingham, UK

Neil Craig, Lecturer in Health Economics, Department of Public Health, University of Glasgow, Glasgow, UK

Tony Dans, Associate Professor, Clinical Epidemiology Unit and Section of Cardiology, College of Medicine, University of the Philippines, Manila, Philippines

Rumona Dickson, Lecturer, University of Liverpool, UK

Anna Donald, Evidence-based Strategies Ltd., London, UK

Vikki Entwistle, Programme Director for Participation in Health Care, Health Services Research Unit, Medical School, University of Aberdeen

David Evans, Dissemination Facilitator, London Region Research and Excellence, London, UK

Cynthia Fraser, Information Scientist, Health Services Research Unit, University of Aberdeen, Aberdeen, UK

Paul Garner, Professor in International Health, International Health Division, Liverpool School of Tropical Medicine, Liverpool, UK

Julie Glanville, Information Service Manager, NHS Centre for Reviews and Dissemination, University of York, York, UK

J A Muir Gray, Programmes Director, UK National Screening Committee. www.nech.nhs.uk/screening

Sian Griffiths, Director of Public Health, Oxfordshire Health Authority, Oxford, UK

Roberto Grilli, Senior Executive, Agenzia Saritaria Regionale, Bologna, Italy

Jeremy Grimshaw, Director, Clinical Epidemiology Programme, Ottawa Health Research Institute, and Head, Center for Best Practice, Institute of Population Health, University of Ottawa, Canada

Gordon Guyatt, Professor of Medicine, Departments of Medicine and Clinical Epidemiology and Biostatistics, McMaster University, Hamilton, Ontario, Canada

Andrew Haines, Dean, London School of Hygiene and Tropical Medicine, London, UK

Margaret Haines, Director of Research and Knowledge Management, NHS Executive South East, London, UK

Emma Harvey, Research Fellow, Department of Health Sciences and Clinical Evaluation, University of York, York, UK

Brian Haynes, Professor and Chair, Department of Clinical Epidemiology and Biostatistics, McMaster University Faculty of Health Sciences, Hamilton, Ontario, Canada

Ellen Hodnett, Professor and Heather M Reisman Chair in Perinatal Nursing Research, University of Toronto, Toronto, Ontario, Canada

Rajendra Kale, Consultant neurologist, Inlaks and Budhrani Hospital Pune, India

R J Lilford, Professor of Clinical Epidemiology, Department of Public Health and Epidemiology, The University of Birmingham, Birmingham, UK

Theresa M Marteau, Professor of Health Psychology, Psychology and Genetics Research Group, King's College, London, UK

Ruairidh Milne, Scientific Director, Wessex Institute for Health Research and Development, Winchester, Southampton, UK

Mary Ann O'Brien, Senior Research Manager, Supportive Cancer Care Research Unit, and Associate Clinical Professor, School of Rehabilitation Science, McMaster University, Hamilton, Ontario, Canada

Graham Mowatt, Research Fellow, Health Services Research Unit, University of Aberdeen, Aberdeen, UK

Sandy Oliver, Research Fellow, Social Science Research Unit, London University Institute of Education, London, UK

Andy Oxman, Director, Health Services Research Unit, National Institute of Public Health, Oslo, Norway

S G Pauker, Professor and Vice Chair, Department of Medicine, New England Medical Center, Tufts University, Boston, Massachusetts, USA

Rodrigo Salinas, Neurologist and Director of the Health Technology Assessement Unit, Ministry of Health, Sarbiago, Chile

Trevor A Sheldon, Professor of Health Studies, University of York, York, UK

Liz Shirran, Research Fellow, Department of General Practice and Primary Care, University of Aberdeen, Aberdeen, UK

Helen Smith, Research Associate, Effective Health Care Alliance Programme, International Health Division, Liverpool School of Tropical Medicine, UK

Vivienne van Someren, Consultant Paediatrician and Senior Lecturer in Child Health, Department of Child Health, Royal Free and University College Medical School, London, UK

Amanda Sowden, Senior Research Fellow, NHS Centre for Reviews and Dissemination, University of York, York, UK

Sharon E Straus, Assistant Professor of Medicine, University Health Network, University of Toronto, Canada

Matthew Sutton, Senior Research Fellow, Department of General Practice, University of Glasgow, Glasgow, UK

Paul Taylor, Lecturer, Centre for Health Informatics and Multiprofessional Education, University College, London, UK

Ruth Thomas, Research Fellow, Health Services Research Unit, Unviersity of Aberdeen, Aberdeen, UK

Jeremy C Wyatt, Reader in Medical Informatics; Director, Knowledge Management Centre, School of Public Policy, University College, London, UK

Lesley Wye, Senior Researcher, King's Fund, London, UK

Foreword

From the beginning one of the main driving forces behind biomedical research, both basic and applied, has been the desire to ultimately improve the health and health services of individuals and communities. Overall, some spectacular advances have been made during the twentieth century; yet it is sometimes said that we would be better off now concentrating on putting into practice what is already known rather than undertaking further research. Of course this would neither be right nor possible since much remains to be learned and it would deny our basic curiosity and inventiveness.

However, the point that is being made concerns the frustration felt by professionals, managers, and policy makers that best practice is not uniformly and universally applied. This is matched by the outrage felt by patients and the public whenever episodes of less than best practice are revealed, a seemingly increasing phenomenon.

This book *Getting Research Findings into Practice*, clearly sets out to tackle this problem head on and is an important contribution to the subject. It recognises the increasing pressure from all concerned to develop more effective dissemination of knowledge into practice. It further recognises that the issues are researchable in their own right and many contributions consider the knowledge base of their topic, often with the depressing conclusion that the studies are not numerous or are flawed methodologically. Readers who are currently in practice will be fascinated by the examples and case studies, which sometimes illustrate dramatically the contrast between success and failure.

But, as the book emphasises, there are no simple answers – if there were, research into practice would not be an issue. The theoretical basis of changing practice needs to be developed. Busy professionals need to know how to access relevant knowledge. Ways of packaging knowledge, including specialist analysis of research findings, need to be improved. Disseminators and the variety of methods at their disposal are important as is a supportive environment. Finally there must be recognition that the application of knowledge must be context dependent and this context might be individual, collective or both.

The theory is challenging, the practice difficult, but *Getting Research Findings into Practice* is both readable and rewarding. The subject will continue to develop and there is no doubt that further editions will be needed and welcomed in due course.

Professor Sir John Pattison
Director of Research, Analysis and Information

1 Introduction

ANDREW HAINES AND ANNA DONALD

Several factors have fuelled ongoing interest in promoting the uptake of research findings. First, in almost all countries there are well documented disparities between clinical practice and research evidence of effective interventions. Examples include secondary prevention of coronary heart disease; management of cardiac failure; atrial fibrillation; asthma; and pregnancy and childbirth.[1-4]

Second, there has been growing awareness of the need to demonstrate that money spent on research and development benefits patients. In the United Kingdom, the advent of the National Health Service (NHS) Research & Development Programme has led to greater involvement of NHS personnel in setting priorities;[5] establishing programmes capable of evaluating different methods of implementing research findings;[6] and assessing the payback on research.[7] Health service users are also increasingly expecting health professionals to demonstrate that they are up to date with advances in knowledge.

Third, there is growing awareness of global trends which will put more and more pressure on health systems to deliver high quality care within tight budgets. These trends include ageing populations; decreasing ratios of workers to dependants in a number of countries until well into the 2030s; and price inflation of medical technologies, which still runs at about double that of other goods and services.

Fourth, there is widespread awareness that passive diffusion of information to keep health professionals up to date is doomed to failure in a global environment in which around two million articles on medical issues are published annually.[8] Most now understand that conventional continuing education activities, such as didactic conferences, courses, and guidelines lacking implementation strategies, have little impact on health professionals' behaviour. Yet health professionals[9] are aware, as never before, of their need to plan for a rapid rate of change in knowledge throughout their lifetimes, which encompasses not only diagnostic techniques, drug therapy, behavioural interventions, and surgical procedures, but also ways of organising and delivering health services.

1

Many health professionals already feel overburdened and undersupported. The challenge remains to find new realistic approaches which enable health professionals to manage change[10] rather than feeling like its victims. A number of steps are necessary.

Keeping abreast of new knowledge

Health professionals need valid and relevant information available at the point of decision making, without appreciable delay. Currently, despite extensive investment in information technology, such information is not widely available. Relatively simple prompting and reminder systems can improve clinicians' performance[11] and prices of useful information sources, such as Clinical Evidence, Best Evidence (which comprises *Evidence based Medicine* and the *American College of Physicians Journal Club* on CD-ROM) and the Cochrane Library are little more than those for journal subscriptions. There are an increasing number of evidence-based journals which summarise important papers in a rigorous fashion and present the results in a way which busy clinicians can rapidly digest. A growing number of organisations, such as the NHS Reviews and Dissemination Centre in York, compile systematic reviews relevant to clinicians and policy makers. While clinicians' access to the Internet is rapidly improving, many clinicians still do not have reliable or timely access to such information,[12] and more needs to be done to provide a wider range of high quality information which is usable in practice settings.

Librarians' roles have undergone enormous change. In North America, for example, some are involved in clinical practice through programmes such as "literature attached to the chart" (LATCH).[13] In such programmes, hospital librarians participate in ward rounds and actively support clinical decision making at the bedside. Requests for information are documented in the notes in the articles, which are subsequently delivered to the ward. Such programmes could be introduced elsewhere with appropriate evaluation, but information support is also needed in primary care, which is still woefully undersupported. Moreover, in the United Kingdom, many health professionals, such as nurses, are still often barred from using library services, as they are not formally affiliated with the medical body that pays for them.

Implementing knowledge

Research findings can influence decisions at many levels – individual patient care; practice guidelines; commissioning of health care and research;

prevention and health promotion; policy development; education; and clinical audit – but only if we know how to translate knowledge into action. Acquiring database searching and critical appraisal skills should give health professionals greater confidence in tracking down and assessing quality of publications, and much attention has been given to the use of electronic information during the consultation with individual patients, using an evidence-based approach derived largely from epidemiological methods. This does not, however, necessarily help them apply new knowledge to day-to-day problems.[14]

First, many decisions require organisational change for their implementation.[15-16] For example, even a step as simple as ensuring that all patients with a past history of myocardial infarction are offered aspirin requires a number of steps to be taken, including identifying the patient; making contact with them; explaining the rationale; checking for contraindications; and prescribing the drug or asking the patient to purchase it over the counter. Furthermore, health professionals have their own experiences, beliefs, and perceptions about appropriate practice. Attempts to change practice which ignore these factors are likely to founder.

This awareness has led to greater emphasis on the understanding of social, behavioural, and organisational factors which may act as barriers to change.[17] Improved understanding requires insight from a number of fields, including education, psychology, sociology, anthropology, information technology, economics, and management studies. A wide spectrum of approaches and interventions for promoting implementation has been used that is underpinned by a number of theoretical perspectives on behaviour change, such as cognitive theories that focus on rational information seeking and decision making; management theories that emphasise organisational conditions needed to improve care; learning theories that lead to behavioural approaches involving, for example, audit and feedback; and reminder systems and social influence theories that focus on understanding and using the social environment to promote and reinforce change.[18]

Responses include increasing attention to quality improvement, particularly to the reduction of medical error rates and the monitoring of healthcare processes and outcomes. In the United Kingdom, concerns about quality improvement have led to "clinical governance", which makes health professionals responsible as never before for the continuous evaluation and improvement of healthcare services. Another innovation, which is being watched by industry, healthcare providers, and governments worldwide, is England's National Institute of Clinical Excellence (NICE), launched in 1999.[28] NICE is a government body charged with evaluating new technologies for clinical and cost effectiveness, and using this information in national purchasing decisions.

Second, it has become increasingly obvious that few practitioners have time or skills to search and appraise all the evidence in their own time. While the number and quality of information resources has increased a great deal during the past few years, few health professionals have all the information they need at their finger-tips during consultations. Information systems, including England's National Electronic Library for Health and *Clinical Evidence* have greatly improved in the past couple of years, and no doubt will continue to develop.

Clearly, these two approaches are not mutually exclusive. For example, the transmission of information derived from research to single practitioners or small groups of health professionals (educational outreach or academic detailing) has a strong educational component but may also include aspects of social influence interventions[19] by, for example, pointing out the use of a particular treatment by local colleagues. The marketing approach used by the pharmaceutical industry to promote its own products depends on segmentation of the target audience into groups that are likely to share characteristics that can be used to tailor the message.[20] Such techniques might be adapted for non-commercial use within the NHS. The evidence for the comparative effectiveness of different approaches and interventions is still patchy and will be reviewed in Chapter 4. It seems likely that in many cases a combination will be more effective than a single intervention.[21] It follows from the above that no single theoretical perspective has been adequately validated to guide the choice of implementation strategies.

The study of the diffusion of innovations, by which new ideas are transmitted through social networks, has been influential in illustrating that those who adopt new ideas early tend to differ in a number of ways from later adopters, for example having more extensive social and professional networks.[22] However, much of the innovations literature has a "pro-innovation" bias with the underlying assumption that innovations are bound to be beneficial. In health care the challenge is to promote the uptake of innovations that have been shown to be effective, to delay the spread of those that have not yet been shown to be effective, and to prevent the uptake of ineffective innovations.[23]

Although a range of actors can promote the uptake of research findings, including policy makers, commissioning authorities, educators, and provider managers, it is by and large clinicians and their patients who implement findings. Having demonstrated a gap between current/desired practice a number of steps need to be taken in order to get research findings into practice (Box 1.1). A number of characteristics of the "message" also need to be considered (Box 1.2) and may influence the degree to which it is taken up in practice.

The choice of key players will be dependent upon the processes to be changed, for example in primary care, nurses and practice administrative

4

Box 1.1   Steps to promoting the uptake of research findings

- Define the appropriate "message", i.e. information to be used.
- Decide which processes need to be altered.
- Involve the key players, i.e. those who will implement change or who are in a position to influence the changes.
- Identify the barriers to change and how to overcome them.
- Decide on specific interventions to promote change, for example guidelines, educational programmes, etc.
- Identify levers for change, i.e. existing mechanisms which can be used to promote change (for example financial incentives to attend educational programmes, placing of appropriate questions in professional examinations).
- Determine whether practice has changed along the desired lines – the use of clinical audit to monitor change.

Box 1.2   Important characteristics of the "message"

Aspects of content:

- Validity
- Generalisability (i.e. settings in which it is relevant)
- Applicability (i.e. patients to whom it is relevant)
- Scope
- Format and presentation (for example written or computerised guidelines; absolute versus relative risk reductions).

Other characteristics:

- Source of the message (for example professional body, Department of Health)
- The channels of communication (i.e. how it is to be disseminated)
- The target audiences (i.e. the recipients)
- Timing of initial launch and frequency of updating
- The mechanism for updating the message.

---

staff should in many cases be involved in addition to the general practitioners, since their cooperation will be essential for effective organisational change. If the innovation involves the acquisition of specific skills, such as training in procedures, then those who organise postgraduate and continuing education are also key players.

Definition of barriers to change and the development of strategies to overcome them are likely to be of key importance in promoting the uptake

5

of research findings. Some examples of barriers to the application of research findings to patients are given in Box 1.3. Chapter 10 proposes a conceptual framework for analysing and overcoming barriers. Since some of the strongest resistance may be related to the experiences and beliefs of health professionals, the early involvement of key players is essential in trying to identify and, where appropriate, overcome such impediments to change.

Box 1.3   Potential barriers to change

These may include:

Practice environment

- Limitations of time
- Practice organisation, for example lack of disease registers or mechanisms to monitor repeat prescribing

Educational environment

- Inappropriate continuing education and failure to link up with programmes to promote quality of care
- Lack of incentives to participate in effective educational activities

Healthcare environment

- Lack of financial resources
- Lack of defined practice populations
- Health policies which promote ineffective or unproven activities
- Failure to provide practitioners with access to appropriate information

Social environment

- Influence of media on patients in creating demands/beliefs
- Impact of disadvantage on patients' access to care

Practitioner factors

- Obsolete knowledge
- Influence of opinion leaders
- Beliefs and attitudes (for example, related to previous adverse experience of innovation)

Patient factors

- Demands for care
- Perceptions/cultural beliefs about appropriate care.

Note: factors which in some circumstances may be perceived as barriers to change can also be levers for change. For example, patients may influence practitioners' behaviour towards clinically effective practice by requesting interventions of proven effectiveness. Practitioners may be influenced positively by opinion leaders.

Interventions to promote change must be tailored to the problem, the audience, and the resources available. For example, educational outreach may be particularly appropriate for updating primary care practitioners in managing specific conditions, because they tend to work alone or in small groups. Guidelines based on research evidence may be developed and endorsed by national professional organisations and adapted for local use as part of clinical audit and educational programmes. Barriers need to be reviewed during the process of implementation as their nature may change as the process develops.

Linking research with practice

There should be closer links between research and practice so that research is relevant to practitioners' needs and practitioners are willing to participate in research. While there is evidence that researchers can be product champions of their work,[24] in general the research community has not been systematically involved in the implementation of their own findings and may not be well equipped to do so. In the United Kingdom, the NHS R&D Programme has made an important start by seeking views about priorities for research through a broad consultation process,[5] but better methods of involving users of research findings are needed to ensure that research questions are appropriately framed and tested in relevant contexts, using interventions that can be replicated in the conditions of day-to-day practice. For example, there is little point conducting trials of a new intervention in hospital practice if virtually all treatments are carried out in primary care settings. Contextual relevance is particularly important for studies of organisation and delivery of services[25] such as stroke units, hospital-at-home schemes, and schemes for improving hospital discharge. If unaccounted for, differences in skill mix and management structures between innovative services and most providers can make it difficult for providers to have a clear view of how they should best implement findings in their own units.

Interaction between purchasers and providers

Purchasers as well as providers should be involved in the application of research findings to practice.[26] Purchasers can help to create an environment that is conducive to change by ensuring that health professionals have access to information, libraries are supported financially, and continuing education and audit programmes are configured to work together to promote effective practice. Purchasers can also ensure that the organisation and delivery of services take into account the best available

7

research evidence. However, it is also clear that the degree of purchaser influence on provider practice is limited[27] and that priority must be given to helping providers to develop the capacity to understand and use evidence.

Making implementation an integral part of training

For many health professionals, involvement in implementation may be far more relevant to their careers and to the development of the NHS than undertaking laboratory research, yet pressures to undertake the latter remain strong. Greater emphasis should be given to encouraging clinicians to spend time learning to use and implement research findings effectively.

Conclusion

Enabling health professionals to evaluate research evidence and to use it in daily practice is an important part of lifelong professional development. This requires not only changes in educational programmes but also a realignment of institutions so that management structures support changes in knowledge and the implementation of changes in procedures.

Currently, there remain major structural difficulties which need to be overcome in the NHS, which everyone is working hard to address. For example better coordination is required between education and training, clinical audit, and research and development. This could be a priority for the National Institute of Clinical Excellence.[28] In addition, it has been suggested that financial considerations rather than potential for learning needs are affecting general practitioners' choice of continuing education courses.[29] Part of continuing education should be directed towards ensuring practitioners keep up with research findings of major importance for patient care and change their practice accordingly. Continuing education activities need to take into account the evidence about the ineffectiveness of many traditional approaches. To overcome fragmentation and develop a more integrated approach for promoting the uptake of research findings, health systems need to develop coordinated mechanisms to deal with the continuing evolution of medical knowledge.

The advent of research-based information[30] for patients and growing accessibility by patients to information of variable quality through the internet and other sources suggest potential for doctors to work as information brokers and interpreters with patients and to work in concert with user groups, a number of which have demonstrated an interest and commitment to providing quality, research-based information to their members.[31] The pace of change in knowledge is unlikely to slow and as health systems around the world struggle to reconcile such change with limited resources and rising expectations, pressure to implement findings of research more effectively and efficiently is bound to grow.

References

1 Campbell NC, Thain J, Deans HG, Ritchie LD, Rawles JM. Secondary prevention in coronary heart disease: baseline survey of provision in general practice. *BMJ* 1998;**316**: 1430–4.
2 Sudlow M, Rodgers H, Kenny R, Thornson R. Population-based study of use of anticoagulants among patients with atrial fibrillation in the community. *BMJ* 1996;**314**:1529–30.
3 Nuffield Institute for Health, University of Leeds, NHS Centre for Reviews and Dissemination, University of York, and Royal College of Physicians Research Unit. The management of menorrhagia. *Effective Health Care Bulletin 9*. Leeds: University of Leeds, 1995.
4 Enkin M. The need for evidence based obstetrics. *Evidence Based Medicine* 1996;**1**:132–3.
5 Jones R, Lamont T, Haines A. Setting priorities for research and development in the NHS: a case study on the interface between primary and secondary care. *BMJ* 1995;**311**:1076–80.
6 Advisory Group to the NHS Central Research and Development Committee. *Methods for the implementation of the findings of research priorities for evaluation*. Leeds: Department of Health, 1995.
7 Buxton M, Hanney S. How can payback from health services' research be assessed? *J Health Serv Res Policy* 1995;**1**:10–18.
8 Mulrow CD. Rationale for systematic reviews. *BMJ* 1994;**309**:597–9.
9 Davis DA, Thomson MA, Oxman AD, Haynes RB. Changing physician performance: a systematic review of continuing medical education strategies. *JAMA* 1995;**274**:700–5.
10 Nuffield Institute for Health, University of Leeds, NHS Centre for Reviews and Dissemination, University of York, and Royal College of Physicians Research Unit. Implementing clinical guidelines. *Effective Health Care Bulletin 8*. Leeds: University of Leeds, 1994.
11 Johnston ME, Langton KB, Haynes RB, Mathiew A. The effects of computer-based clinical decision support systems on clinician performance and patients' outcome. A critical appraisal of research. *Ann Intern Med* 1994;**120**:135–42.
12 Prescott K, Douglas HR, Lloyd M, Haines A, Rosenthal J, Watt G. General Practitioners' awareness of and attitudes towards research-based information. *Fam Pract* 1997;**14**:320–3.
13 Cimpl K. Clinical medical librarianship: a review of the literature. *Bull Med Libr Assoc* 1985;**73**:21–8.
14 Hyde CJ. Using the evidence. A need for quantity, not quality. *Int J Assess Health Care* 1996;**12**(2):280–7.
15 Sackett DL, Haynes RB, Rosenberg W, Haynes RB. *Evidence-based medicine: how to practice and teach ERM*. London: Churchill Livingstone, 1997.
16 Evidence-based Medicine Working Group. Evidence-based medicine. A new approach to teaching the practice of medicine. *JAMA* 1992;**268**:2420–5.
17 Oxman A, Flotorp S. An overview of strategies to promote implementation of evidence based health care. In: Silagy C, Haines A (ed.) *Evidence-Based Practice in Primary Care*. London; BMJ Books, 1998.
18 Grol R. Beliefs and evidence in changing clinical practice. *BMJ* 1997;**315**:418–21.
19 Mittman BS, Tonesk X, Jacobson PD. Implementing clinical practice guidelines: social influence strategies and practitioner behaviour change. *Qual Rev Bull* 1992;**18**:413–21.
20 Lidstone J. *Market planning for the pharmaceutical industry*. Aldershot: Gower, 1987.
21 Oxman A, Davis D, Haynes RB, Ihornson MA. No magic bullets: a systematic review of 102 trials of interventions to help health professionals deliver services more effectively or efficiently. *Can Med Assoc J* 1995;**153**:1423–43.

22 Rogers EM. *Diffusion of innovations.* New York: Free Press, 1983.
23 Haines A, Jones R. Implementing findings of research. *BMJ* 1994;**308**:1488–92.
24 Gouws D. ed. *Case studies with a view to implementation.* Pretoria, South Africa: Human Sciences Research Council, 1994.
25 Haines A, Iliffe S. Innovations in services and the appliance of science. *BMJ* 1995;**310**: 875–6.
26 Evans D, Haines A, eds. *Implementing evidence-based changes in health care* Abingdon UK: Radcliffe Medical Press, 2000.
27 Hopkins A, Solomon JK. Can contracts drive clinical care? *BMJ* 1996;**313**:477–8.
28 Secretary of State for Health. *The new NHS: modern, dependable.* London: The Stationery Office, 1997.
29 Murray TS, Campbell LM. Finance, not learning needs, makes general practitioners attend courses: a database survey. *BMJ* 1997;**315**:353.
30 Stocking B. Partners in care. *Health Man* 1997;**1**:12–13.
31 Stocking B. Implementing the findings of effective care in pregnancy and childbirth. *Milbank Q* 1993;**71**:497–522.

2 Criteria for the implementation of research evidence in policy and practice

TREVOR A SHELDON, GORDON GUYATT, AND ANDREW HAINES

Key messages

- Evidence of net benefit should be assessed by the evaluation of the methods used in different studies.
- The evidence should be put into perspective.
- The applicability of the research to practice settings should be assessed.
- Priorities should be set for implementation.

Introduction

There is increasing interest in "evidence based health care" where decisions made by healthcare professionals, provider management, purchasers, healthcare commissioners, the public, and policy makers consistently consider research evidence.[1-3] Purchasers, for example, should be able to influence the organisation and delivery of care, such as for cancer,[4] the organisation of stroke services,[5] and the type and content of services (such as chiropractic for back pain[6] or dilatation and curettage for menorrhagia).[7] Policy makers should ensure that policy is consistent with evidence, that the incentive structure within the health system promotes cost-effective practice, and that there is an adequate infrastructure for producing, gathering, summarising, and disseminating evidence and for monitoring changes in practice. Clinicians determine the day-to-day care patients receive in healthcare systems and user groups are also beginning to play an important role in influencing broad healthcare decisions.[8]

This chapter outlines the factors that should be considered when deciding whether to act upon, or to promote the implementation of, the findings of research.

Convincing evidence of net benefit

Evaluating the methods of primary studies

Individual research studies vary in the degree to which they are likely to mis-estimate the effectiveness of an intervention (bias). Observational studies, in which investigators compare the results of groups of patients receiving different treatments according to clinicians' or patients' preferences, are susceptible to bias because the prognosis of the groups is likely to differ in unpredictable ways, leading to spuriously reduced or, more commonly, inflated treatment effects.

Rigorous randomised controlled trials, by ensuring that the groups being compared are indeed similar, greatly reduce bias.[9] As long as patients are analysed in the groups to which they are randomised, this process permits a more confident inference that the treatments offered are responsible for differences in outcome. Randomised controlled trials are useful not only for testing the effectiveness of interventions in tightly controlled clinical settings but also across a wide spectrum of health research.[10,11] Inference is further strengthened if patients, care givers, and those assessing outcomes are blind to allocation to treatment or control and if follow-up is complete.[12]

Whilst randomised controlled trials are often regarded as the gold standard for comparing the efficacy of treatments, other study designs are appropriate for evaluating other types of healthcare technologies and factors such as potentially harmful exposures, and indicators of prognosis.[13] Increasingly, qualitative methods are being used, for example to provide an understanding of patients' and professionals' attitudes, behaviours, situations, and their interactions.[14]

Whatever the appropriate design, practitioners will often discover that research evidence is biased or otherwise limited; for example, the investigators may have focused on inappropriate end-points, such as physiological measures, rather than outcomes of relevance to patients.[15] Particularly in evaluations of healthcare organisation, providers must consider whether treatment effects were really due to the putative intervention. For example, in positive randomised controlled trials evaluating stroke units, was the impact due to the organisational structure or to the greater skill or enthusiasm of those who established the unit?[5] Uncertainty about the magnitude and direction of treatment effects may be heightened by small sample sizes, leading to wide confidence intervals. Though practitioners will still need to make use of imperfect research information, new clinical policies should rarely be implemented unless clinicians find strong evidence for benefit.

Evaluating the methods of overviews of groups of studies

Systematic overviews can provide reliable summaries of data addressing targeted clinical questions, and less biased estimates of treatment effects[16] if they adhere to the criteria shown in Box 2.1.[17,18]

Evaluating the results of systematic overviews

A rigorous systematic overview may leave the decision maker uncertain. First, the primary studies may be methodologically weak. Second, unexplained variability between study results may leave doubt about whether to believe studies showing larger treatment effects or those showing no benefit. Third, even after pooling results across studies, small sample size may leave the confidence intervals wide. Thus the research evidence may be consistent with a large, or a negligible, treatment effect. Fourth, because of the side-effects associated with a treatment, or the cost, the trade-off between treating and not treating may be precarious. Classifications of the strength of research evidence supporting use of a particular treatment should consider each of these four issues. For example, grades of strength of evidence of treatment effectiveness have been developed on methodological grounds using the type and quality of study design and the variability of study results.[19] Thus for example, a systematic review of randomised controlled trials which show consistent results (such as trials of streptokinase for treatment of acute myocardial infarction)[3] would be regarded as higher quality evidence than a review of randomised controlled trials which show variable results (heterogeneity) without good explanation. We could further consider the precision of the estimated treatment effect and the trade-off between the benefits and risks. In making the latter assessment, we must note that many studies of efficacy, and overviews of these studies, do not

---

Box 2.1   Criteria to increase reliability of a systematic review

- Use of explicit inclusion and exclusion criteria, including specification of the population, the intervention, the outcome, and the methodological criteria for the studies they include
- Comprehensive search methods used to locate relevant studies
- Assessment of the validity of the primary studies
- Assessment of the primary studies that is reproducible and attempts to avoid bias
- Exploration of variation between the study findings
- Appropriate synthesis and, when suitable, pooling of primary studies

provide sufficient information of the possible harm (such as side-effects) of treatments. Randomised trials are usually not large or long enough to detect rare or long-term harmful effects.[20] Large observational studies may be useful in determining the probability of harm.[21]

Putting evidence of benefit into perspective

Evidence of effectiveness does not imply that an intervention should be adopted; this depends on whether the benefit is sufficiently large relative to the risks and costs. For example, the small positive effect of beta interferon in the treatment of multiple sclerosis relative to the cost leaves implementation questionable.[22,23]

One approach to the decision to implement an intervention is to determine a threshold above which one would routinely offer treatment and below which one would not. Decision makers can consider the threshold, for example in terms of the number of patients one would need to treat to prevent a single adverse event (such as a death).[24] The threshold "number needed to treat" defines the value above which the disadvantages of treatment outweigh the benefits (and treatment may therefore be withheld) and below which the benefits outweigh the disadvantages (and treatment may therefore be offered).[25] Because treatments vary with respect to their costs and their effects on length and quality of life, each intervention would need a separate threshold "number needed to treat", which will also vary according to the values of the patient or population being offered the intervention.

Where reliable data is available, a threshold might be expressed in terms of a cost-effectiveness ratio giving the cost of achieving a unit of benefit (for example quality-adjusted life year, taking into account equity factors) below which an intervention is seen as worth routinely implementing. Quantitative research evidence inevitably is probabilistic and subject to various forms of uncertainty and is rarely the sole basis of decision making at governmental or the clinical level. Indeed, uncertainty is one obstacle to policy makers using research evidence.[26] Differences in people's risk averseness is one explanation for variations in decision making in the face of the same evidence. However, research evidence should play an important and arguably greater part in decision making and can provide a benchmark against which decisions may be audited.

Applicability of the research to practice settings

The decision as to whether the research evidence can or should be applied in relation to a specific patient cannot always be simply translated from the research. Results of evaluative studies are usually in the form of average effects. Patients may differ from the average, however, in ways which

14

Box 2.2   Factors to consider when applying research evidence to individual patients

- Is the relative risk reduction due to the intervention likely to be different because of the patient's physiological or clinical characteristics?
- What is the patient's absolute risk of an adverse event without intervention?
- Is there significant co-morbidity or contraindication which may reduce benefit?
- Are there social or cultural factors, for example, that might affect treatment suitability or acceptability?
- What do the patient and their family want?

---

influence the effectiveness of the treatment (relative risk reduction) or the impact (absolute risk reduction).[27,28] Box 2.2 summarises factors which clinicians and patients should consider before applying research evidence.

The sorts of patients who participate in trials may not be typical of the types of the people for whom the treatment is potentially useful.[29] However, it is probably more appropriate to assume that research findings are generalisable across patients unless there is strong theoretical or empirical evidence to suggest that a particular patient group will respond differently.[27] There may, however, be a heterogeneity of effect across patients because of biological, social, and other differences that influence the effect of the intervention or the level of risk of an adverse outcome.[29,30] For example, beta blockers may be less effective than diuretics at reducing blood pressure in black people of African descent than in white populations.[31] Interventions are more likely to impact uniformly on the population where the situation is closer to a purely biological process in which there is low variation within the population than when many patient-specific and contextual factors intervene.[32] These issues are important when targeting "effective" treatments for disadvantaged groups with the aim of reducing inequalities in health. If, for example, smoking cessation interventions are less successful in poorer groups then an anti-smoking programme might not have the anticipated effects on equity.

In a large number of chronic conditions, including chronic pain syndromes (such as arthritis from treatment) or chronic heart or lung disease where benefit may vary widely between individual patients, single-patient randomised controlled trials (N-of-1 RCTs) may help to determine a particular patient's response to treatment.[33]

Clinicians must give particular consideration to patients in whom treatment may be contraindicated or where there is substantial co-morbidity. In the latter case, a reduction of the risk of dying from one disease might not reduce overall risk of dying because of risk of a competing cause of death.

15

The effect of an intervention may also vary because patients do not share the same morbidity or risk.[34] For any given level of treatment effectiveness, patients at higher levels of risk will generally experience greater levels of absolute risk reduction or impact.[30,34–36] For example, patients at high risk of death from coronary heart disease treated with cholesterol-lowering drugs will experience a greater reduction in mortality risk than those at lower risk – we might have to treat 30 high-risk patients for five years to save a life, but 300 low-risk patients.[17,37,38] Thus, what might be worth implementing in a high-risk patient may not be worth it for a lower-risk patient.[37–39]

The decision to use a treatment will also depend on patient-specific factors. Clinicians will find research studies which consider a range of important outcomes of treatment more useful than those which have only measured a few narrow clinical end-points. More qualitative research within robust quantitative study design will help practitioners and patients better understand and apply the results of research.

Setting priorities

Implementation of research evidence is rarely widespread without concerted attempts to get results into practice.[40,41] It is impossible to promote actively the implementation of the results of all systematic reviews because of the limited capacity of healthcare systems to absorb new research and the investment necessary to overcome obstacles to getting research into practice.[41] These costs must be considered in relation to the likely payback in terms of health improvements. The anticipated benefits of implementation will vary according to factors such as the divergence between research evidence and current practice or policies that influence the marginal benefit of further implementation efforts.

When faced with the same evidence, different classes of decision makers may have different criteria for choosing priorities for implementation. For example, policy makers look more for societal gains in health and efficiency while for clinicians the well-being of their patients is of prime importance.[42] Formal decision analysis may be helpful for setting priorities for implementation and in applying research evidence with individual patients.[43,44]

The degree to which clinicians see even good quality research as implementable will depend on whether they have the relevant skills and the extent to which the results conflict with professional experience and cherished beliefs. This reflects an epistemological mismatch between the sort of evidence researchers produce and believe and the sort of evidence practising clinicians value.[45] The implications of research evidence for policy and practice are often not straightforward or obvious[46] and this ambiguity may result in the same evidence giving rise to divergent conclusions and action.[47] Many clinicians and policy makers will prefer to await confirmatory evidence, depending on the perceived risks, the extent of change required, and the

16

quality and certainty of the research results. When designing studies, investigators should think how and by whom their results will be used. The design should be sufficiently robust, the setting sufficiently similar to that in which the results are likely to be implemented, the outcomes should be relevant, and the study size large enough for the results to convince decision makers.

References

1 Davidoff F, Haynes RB, Sackett D, Smith R. Evidence based medicine [editorial]. *BMJ* 1995;**310**:1122–6.
2 Guyatt GH. Evidence based medicine [editorial]. *ACP J Club* 1991;A–16.
3 Antman EM, Lau J, Kupelnick B, Mosteller F, Chalmers TC. A comparison of the results of controlled trials and recommendations of clinical experts. Treatments for myocardial infarction. *JAMA* 1992;**268**:240–8.
4 *NHS Executive guidance for purchasers: Improving outcomes in breast cancer – the manual* (96CC0021). London: Department of Health, 1996.
5 Stroke Unit Trialists' Collaboration. A systematic review of specialist multidisciplinary (stroke unit) care for stroke in patients. In: Warlow C, van Gijn J, Sandercock P. ed. *Stroke module of the Cochrane Database of Systematic Reviews*. London: BMJ Publishing Group, 1997.
6 Shekelle P. *Spinal manipulation and mobilisation for low back pain*. Paper presented at the International Forum for Primary Care Research on Low Back Pain, Seattle, October 1995.
7 NHS Centre for Reviews and Dissemination; University of York. Management of menorrhagia. *Effective Health Care Bulletin* 1995;**1**(9).
8 Entwistle V, Sheldon TA, Sowden A, Watt I. Evidence-informed patient choice: issues of involving patients in decisions about health care technologies. *Int J Tech Assess Health Care* 1998;**14**:212–25.
9 Schultz K, Chalmers I, Haynes RJ, Altman DG. Empirical evidence of bias. Dimensions of methodological quality associated with estimates of treatment effects in controlled clinical trials. *JAMA* 1995;**273**:408–12.
10 Green SB. The eating patterns study – the importance of practical randomized trials in communities. *Am J Public Health* 1997;**87**:541–3.
11 Bauman KE. The effectiveness of family planning programs evaluated with true experimental designs. *Am J Public Health* 1997;**87**:666–9.
12 Guyatt GH, Sackett DL, Cook DJ, for the evidence based medicine working group. Users' guide to the medical literature. II. How to use an article about therapy or prevention. Part A – Are the results valid? *JAMA* 1993;**270**:2598–601.
13 Laupacis A, Wells G, Richardson WS, Tugwell P, for the evidence based medicine working group. Users' guides to the medical literature. V. How to use an article about prognosis. *JAMA* 1994;**272**:234–7.
14 Mays N, Pope C. *Qualitative research in health care*. London: BMJ Publishing Group, 1996.
15 Gotzche PC, Liberati A, Torri V, Rossetti L. Beware of surrogate end-points. *Int J Tech Assess Health Care* 1996;**12**:238–46.
16 Chalmers I, Altman D. *Systematic reviews*. London: BMJ Publishing Group, 1995.
17 Oxman AD, Cook DJ, Guyatt GH, for the evidence based medicine working group. Users' guide to the medical literature. VI. How to use an overview. *JAMA* 1993;**272**:1367–71.
18 *Undertaking systematic reviews of research on effectiveness. CRD guidelines for those carrying out or commissioning reviews*. CRD Report 4. University of York: NHS Centre for Reviews and Dissemination, 1996.
19 Liddle J, Williamson M, Irwig L. *Method for evaluating research and guidelines evidence*. Sydney: NSW Health Department, 1996.
20 Levine M, Walter S, Lee H, Haines T, Holbrook A, Moyer V, for the evidence based medicine working group. Users' guides to the medical literature. IV. How to use an article about harm. *JAMA* 1994;**271**:1615–19.

21 Palareti G, Leali N, Coccher S, et al. Bleeding complications of oral anticoagulant treatment: an inception-cohort, prospective collaborative study (ISCOAT). Lancet 1996;**348**;423–8.
22 Walley T, Barton S. A purchaser perspective of managing new drugs: interferon beta as a case study. BMJ 1995;**311**:796–9.
23 Rous E, Coppel A, Haworth J, Noyce S. A purchaser experience of managing new expensive drugs: interferon beta. BMJ 1996;**313**:1195–6.
24 Cook RJ, Sackett DL, The number needed to treat – a clinically useful measure of treatment. BMJ 1995;**310**:452–4.
25 Guyatt GH, Sackett DL, Sinclair JC et al. Users' guide to the medical literature. IX. A method for grading health care recommendations. JAMA 1995;**274**:1800–4.
26 Hammond K, Mumpower J, Dennis RL, Fitch S, Crumpacker W. Fundamental obstacles to the use of scientific information in public policy making. Technological Forecasting and Social Change 1983;**24**:287–97.
27 Davis CE. Generalizing from clinical trials. Controlled Clinical Trials 1994;**15**:11–14.
28 Wittes RE. Problems in the medical interpretation of overviews. Stats in Med 1987;**6**:269–76.
29 Pearson TA, Myers M. Treatment of hypercholesterolemia in women: equality, effectiveness, and extrapolation of evidence. JAMA 1997;**277**:1320–1.
30 Bailey KR. Generalizing the results of randomized clinical trials. Controlled Clinical Trials 1994;**15**:15–23.
31 Veterans Administration Cooperative Study Group. Comparison of propranolol and hydrochlorothiazide for the initial treatment of hypertension. 1: Results of short-term titration with emphasis on racial differences in response. JAMA 1982;**248**:1996–2003.
32 Cowan CD, Wittes J. Intercept studies, clinical trials, and cluster experiments: to whom can we extrapolate? Controlled Clinical Trials 1994;**15**:24–9.
33 Mahon J, Laupacis A, Donner A, Wood T. Randomised study of N-of-1 trials versus standard practice. BMJ 1996;**312**:1069–74.
34 Davey Smith G, Eggar M. Who benefits from medical interventions? BMJ 1993;**308**:72–4.
35 Glasziou PP, Irwig LM. An evidence based approach to individualising treatment. BMJ 1995;**311**:356–9.
36 Oxman AD, Guyatt GH. A consumer's guide to subgroup analysis. Ann Intern Med 1992;**116**:78–84.
37 Davey Smith G, Song F, Sheldon TA. Cholesterol lowering and mortality: the importance of considering initial level of risk. BMJ 1993;**306**:1367–73.
38 Marchioli R, Marfisi RM, Carinci F, Tognoni G. Meta-analysis, clinical trials, and transferability of research results into practice. Arch Intern Med 1996;**156**:1158–72.
39 Ramsey LE, Haq IU, Jackson PR, Yeo WW, Pickin DM, Payne N. Targeting lipid-lowering drug therapy for primary prevention of coronary disease: an updated Sheffield table. Lancet 1996;**348**:387–8.
40 Oxman A, Davis D, Haynes RB, Thomson MA. No magic bullets: a systematic review of 102 trials of interventions to help health professionals deliver services more effectively and efficiently. Can Med Assoc J 1995;**153**:1423–43.
41 Haines A, Jones R. Implementing findings of research. BMJ 1994;**308**:1488–92.
42 Diamond GA, Denton TA. Alternative perspectives on the biased foundation of medical technology assessment. Ann Intern Med 1993;**118**:455–64.
43 Thornton JG, Lilford RJ. Decision analysis for managers. BMJ 1995;**310**:791–4.
44 Lilford RJ, Thornton JG. Decision logic in medical practice. J Royal Coll Phys 1992;**26**:400–12.
45 Tanenbaum SJ. Knowing and acting in medical practice: the epistemological politics of outcomes research. J Health Politics and Law 1994;**19**:27–44.
46 Naylor CD. Grey zones of clinical practice: some limits to evidence based medicine. Lancet 1995;**345**:840–2.
47 Tanenbaum SJ. "Medical effectiveness" in Canadian and US health policy: the comparative politics of inferential ambiguity. Health Serv Res 1996;**31**:517–32.

3 Sources of information on clinical effectiveness and methods of dissemination

JULIE GLANVILLE, MARGARET HAINES, AND IONE AUSTON

> **Key messages**
> - Practice should be based on good quality systematic reviews and other high quality research.
> - Many resources are already available for clinicians to use.
> - Strategies for finding and filtering information are available.
> - Improvements to dissemination practices are required so that relevant material can be more easily identified.

Introduction

There is increasing pressure on healthcare professionals to ensure that their practice is based on evidence from good quality research such as well conducted randomised controlled trials or preferably systematic reviews of these and other research designs. This pressure comes from several directions. The evidence-based healthcare movement is encouraging a questioning and reflective approach to clinical practice alongside an emphasis on lifelong learning. This relies on good access to research-based evidence. Governments are encouraging the development of evidence-based medicine as they see its advantages in terms of improved efficiency in the delivery of health care through the identification of effective and cost-effective treatments that contribute to a quality service.[1-3]

In addition there are indications that legal decisions may start to take account of adherence to research evidence and clinical guidelines.[4,5] Another incentive for clinicians to be more aware of research will come from better informed consumers. The *NHS Plan* published in 2000 outlines plans for increased British public access to high quality information on treatments and preventive health care.[6] In the United States, MEDLINEplus, the National Library of Medicine's (NLM) consumer health web site, launched in October 1998, is now used by consumers and health professionals throughout the world some 1·3 million times each month.[7] NLM has also started a programme of electronic health information projects aimed at people who do not have access to the internet.[8] Today's clinician needs to be able to access information on clinical effectiveness in order to improve the quality of care and to stay well informed on specialist areas of health care. This chapter examines the issues of access to research-based evidence from three perspectives:

- resources that are already available for clinicians to use
- further strategies for finding and filtering information
- improvements to dissemination practices so that relevant material can be more easily identified.

What evidence-based information is currently available?

In the 1990s great progress was made in making evidence from research more easily available. In part this was achieved through the development of programmes of health technology assessment and, in particular, the growth of systematic reviews. Systematic reviews evaluate the available primary evidence and indicate the effectiveness of particular interventions. A valuable compilation of reviews is available in the Cochrane Library and many reports examining the cost and clinical effectiveness of treatments and ways of organising health care have been published by technology assessment agencies such as the Agency for Healthcare Research and Quality (AHRQ) in the United States and the English Health Technology Assessment Programme. The publications and databases listed in Box 3.1 present evidence on effectiveness, often in a summarised or digested form suitable for the busy clinician or policy maker. However, key problems remain: how to increase awareness of what information is available and how to provide clinicians with information at the time that they need it.

Collections of systematic reviews and critical appraisals of primary research provide valuable access to evaluated research. Inevitably, the proliferation of these collections has created its own information explosion which needs to be addressed in its turn. There is currently no single comprehensive index to all the material described in Box 3.1 so several searches in paper and electronic services may be required to locate relevant information. On the positive side, increasingly the full text of evidence reports is available via the internet and there are many initiatives in progress to provide coherent and structured access to quality assessed collections of evidence, such as the planned 'knowledge floor' of the National Electronic Library for Health (NeLH).[9]

Most of the resources in Box 3.1 provide evaluated and filtered information, i.e. they highlight the best quality studies from the mass of available literature. However, research-based answers to many effectiveness questions are not yet available in such time-saving, value-added forms. Searchers may still need to search indexes and abstracts of the published literature. MEDLINE can be searched on the internet using the PubMed interface which provides access to a mass of peer-reviewed but largely unsynthesised and unevaluated studies. However, PubMed also offers tools to help searchers to identify the types of studies that are more likely to provide high quality information on clinical effectiveness, such as systematic reviews or randomised controlled trials.[10,11] Based on optimal MEDLINE search strategies developed by Brian Haynes and colleagues at McMaster University, PubMed also features a specialised search called Clinical Queries to help busy clinicians quickly retrieve sound clinical studies on the etiology, prognosis, diagnosis, prevention, or treatment of disorders.[12] Once the original papers have been obtained there are checklists which, complemented by critical appraisal skills training, can be used to assess the rigour and validity of such studies.[13]

Although MEDLINE is a rich resource, increasingly access is required to a wider range of material than it presently indexes. The HSTAT service offers access to full text evidence reports, guidelines and guidance.[14] Other databases covering specific clinical areas, specific types of publication, and non-English material also need to be more widely explored. Tools such as search strategies and single interfaces, such as the NLM Gateway or the NeLH, are required that will enhance access to a range of such databases.

Other strategies for finding and filtering information

Training and practice are required to search information services and to navigate the internet and organisation-wide intranets effectively. Locating, appraising, and exploiting subject resources, both print and electronic, has typically been the role of library and information professionals and it has been shown that librarians are often more effective than physicians, particularly trained librarians compared to untrained physicians, in quality filtering of the literature.[15,16] Clinicians are therefore increasingly turning to librarians for assistance in developing these information skills and librarians are now expected to be facilitators, trainers and intranet content managers.[17–19]

However, some physicians simply do not have the time to take up the training being offered or to develop the necessary level of searching competence. They want librarians to continue to provide assistance in

Box 3.1   Selected resources providing summaries or assessments of the effectiveness of interventions

The Cochrane Library

A collection of databases, including the full text of Cochrane Reviews, critical commentaries on selected quality-assessed systematic reviews produced by the NHS Centre for Reviews and Dissemination, records of health technology assessments and brief details of more than 300 000 randomised controlled trials. Details: Update Software, Summertown Pavilion, Middle Way, Summertown, Oxford OX2 7LG.
For details of internet access see http://www.update-software.com/cochrane/cochrane-frame.html

Agency for Healthcare Research and Quality (AHRQ) evidence reports

A series of evidence reports based on thorough reviews of the research evidence. With the American Medical Association and the American Association of Health Plans, AHRQ have also developed an on-line practice guidelines clearinghouse that provides objective summary comparisons of current clinical guidelines. Details: Evidence report summaries available at http://www.ahrq.gov/clinic and in full text at http://text.nlm.nih.gov/. Guideline clearinghouse available at http://www.guideline.gov/

Best Evidence 5 database

Brings together abstracts (published in *ACP Journal Club* and *Evidence based Medicine*) of quality-assessed primary and review articles with a commentary by clinical experts. Details: (1) Website URL: http://www.bmjpg.com; (2) The CD-ROM is available from BMJ Publishing, BMA House, Tavistock Square, London WC1H 9JR.

Effective Health Care Bulletins

Reports of systematic reviews presented in a readable and accessible format. Produced by the NHS Centre for Reviews and Dissemination. Details: Available full text at http://www.york.ac.uk/inst/crd/ehcb.htm. Subscription details are also available at that site.

Clinical Evidence

Evidence-based answers to primary care questions relating to prevention and treatment. Updated every six months. Further information: http://www.clinicalevidenceonline.org

Bandolier

UK newsletter alerting readers to key evidence about healthcare effectiveness. Details: URL http://www.jr2.ox.ac.uk/bandolier/

continued

Box 3.1 *(continued)*

Drug and Therapeutics Bulletin

Independent assessments of drugs and other modes of treatment. Details: Consumers' Association, Castlemead, Gascoyne Way, Hertford SG14 ILH. URL: http://www.which.net/health/dtb/main.html

Effectiveness Matters

Summaries of published research on a single topic pointing out clear effectiveness messages. Details: NHS Centre for Reviews and Dissemination, University of York, York Y01 5DD. URL: http://www.york.ac.uk/inst/crd/em.htm

Health Evidence Bulletins Wales

Evidence-based summaries of treatments in broad disease area, such as mental health, cancers and injury prevention. URL: http://hebw.uwcm.ac.uk/

HSTAT (Health Services Technology Assessment Text)

Full-text resource developed and maintained by the National Library of Medicine containing AHRQ evidence reports and guidelines, the US Task Force on Preventive Services' Guide to Clinical Preventive Services, and other related evidence-based publications. URL: http://text.nlm.nih.gov

NHS Economic Evaluation Database

Critical assessments of published economic evaluations, produced by the NHS Centre for Reviews and Dissemination. Details: URL: http://www.york.ac.uk/inst/crd.

TRIP index

Easy to search index to a large collection of internet-based clinical effectiveness resources. URL: http://www.tripdatabase.com/

Netting the evidence

Collection of links to tools, resources, and guides informing the practice of evidence-based healthcare. URL: http://www.nettingtheevidence.org.uk

---

finding information to answer a particular clinical issue but in a way which is closer to the place and time of need.[20–22] New models have emerged for delivering library support directly to the hospital wards and departments.[23,24] In the United States, the National Network of Libraries of Medicine provide outreach services to general practitioners (and, more recently, to public health professionals) and in the UK the British Medical Association Library also offers an electronic outreach service to members.[25-27] In the UK, the Oxford Primary Care Sharing the Evidence (PRISE) project has explored another model whereby GPs' computers are linked into a central information server computer which provides a range of useful databases and searchers can also request librarians to follow up particular questions in more detail.[28]

An innovative library service has been developed at the Eskind Biomedical Library at Vanderbilt University as part of their Clinical Medical Librarian programme. After extensive in-depth training, librarians at Vanderbilt become part of eight clinical teams. The librarians are full participants, providing not only quality searching and filtering of the medical literature, but also synthesizing highly relevant passages from medical journals into concise informative summaries that they orally present along with articles to their teams during hospital rounds.[29]

Multidisciplinary teams of librarians, clinicians and informatics specialists are also developing clinical decision support software and information filtering systems for internet resources based on user interest profiles, some of which link knowledge resources directly to electronic patient records.[30-33] The University of Washington's MINDscape interface service has librarians working with clinical informatics teams to bring quality information (such as drug reference information, laboratory reference information, and locally reviewed and relevant clinical guidelines) to the wards by integrating these knowledge sources into the University's computer-based medical record system.[34]

The training of librarians will need to change to reflect the new range of skills required in these expanded "knowledge management" roles. This includes developing their technical information management and technology skills, their understanding of the "business" processes of their organisations as well as their capacity for lifelong learning, initiative, assertiveness, flexibility and proactivity.[35,36] Clearly, initiatives such as the Oxford Health Libraries' training programme "Librarian of the Twenty-First Century" and the STRAP programme in the South East region of the NHS are models for other library networks in the UK.[37,38] On the macro level similar efforts to expand the training and education of librarians in the US are being led by the Medical Library Association and the National Library of Medicine. On a micro level there are many other developments to enhance librarian skills. One example is the work of Ann McKibbon and her librarian colleagues at McMaster University in Canada, who have developed a self-study text on evidence-based principles and practice. This is used to train information specialists for effective retrieval of clinically relevant studies and to analyse and interpret the statistical measures on which the study results are based.[39]

The value of investing in developing the role of library and information professionals is supported by studies which have shown that library support not only contributes to lower patient costs through decreased admissions, length of stay, and procedures but also contributes to higher quality of care in terms of patient advice, improved decision making, and time saving.[40,41]

How can researchers, publishers, and information/providers improve dissemination?

This chapter has looked at strategies to locate research-based information. For information to be accessible it must not only be recorded in "popular" sites, but also be packaged and published in formats that promote easy identification and encourage use. Evidence-based information is becoming easier to spot: structured abstracts attached to journal articles are making it easier to identify the methodology and so potentially the reliability of the study. Innovations such as the *BMJ's* key messages box make it easier to identify the key points to be drawn from the research. Journal editors have an important role in encouraging informative abstracts and ensuring that researchers' conclusions are supported by a paper's results. However, the benefits of clearer labelling may be undermined if current "buzzwords" such as "effective" and "evidence-based" are adopted and used incorrectly or inaccurately: previously useful labels may become unhelpful.

Bodies producing policy and clinical recommendations, including guidelines, are finding it necessary to make them more explicitly evidence-based, both in using the available research evidence and in stating the level of evidence on which the guidelines are based. Identifying and appraising the quality of guidelines is being assisted by major developments such as the National Guidelines Clearinghouse developed by the US Agency for Healthcare Research and Quality. This initiative provides summary side-by-side comparisons of clinical practice guidelines based on standard criteria.[42] In the UK St George's Medical School has developed a guideline appraisal tool and presents a collection of appraised guidelines on its web site.[43]

Information from research needs to be presented in appropriate forms for its target audience. The AHRQ guidelines have shown how information can be packaged in different ways for different groups of users by using three levels of publication: a detailed report of the review with a full exposition of the research evidence, a briefer guideline for the clinician, and a leaflet for the patient. In the UK, the Informed Choice leaflets have shown how different leaflets aimed at pregnant women and their professional carers can be produced, based on evidence taken where possible from Cochrane reviews.[44,45]

Improving timely access to information is only one aspect of the implementation of research-based information. Simply presenting research evidence to the clinician is often not sufficient to ensure its incorporation into practice. Even when findings are packaged, summarised, and made relevant to clinicians, further action is needed to ensure their implementation. However, there is now a large research base on how to disseminate research findings and to encourage implementation. Creating this knowledge has been the focus of much primary research, as well as systematic review efforts by the Cochrane Effective Practice and Organization of Care group.[46-48] These research findings around effective dissemination and implementation strategies have also been repackaged to reach yet wider audiences.[49] As we face increasing encouragement to implement clinical guidance and other quality measures, the results of this important work are now more easily accessible to inform efforts to achieve widespread uptake.

References

1 *Priorities and planning guidance for the NHS 1997–1998.* Leeds: Department of Health, NHS Executive, 1996.
2 Glasziou P. Support for trials of promising medications through the Pharmaceutical Benefits Scheme. A proposal for a new authority category. *Med J Aust* 1995;**162**:33–6.
3 Secretary of State for Health. *The new NHS: modern, dependable.* London: Stationery Office, 1997.
4 Tingle J. Developing clinical guidelines: present and future legal aspects. *Br J Nurs* 1998;7(11):672–4.
5 Doctors in the dock. *Economist* 1995(Aug 19):23–4.
6 *The NHS plan: a plan for investment, a plan for reform.* London: Stationery Office, 2000.
7 Extensive drug information added to MEDLINEplus. *NLM Newsline* 2000;**55**(2):1.
8 National Library of Medicine to help consumers use online health data. *JAMA* 2000;**283**(13):1675.
9 National Electronic Library for Health. http://www.nelh.nhs.uk/default.asp (accessed 16 July 2001).
10 Dickersin K, Scherer R, Lefebvre C. Identifying relevant studies for systematic reviews. *BMJ* 1994;**309**:1286–91.
11 McKibbon K, Wilczynski NL, Walker-Dilks Q. How to search for and find evidence about therapy. *Evidence based Medicine*;1(3):70–2.
12 The US National Library of Medicine. PubMed clinical queries using research methodology filters [3 screens]. http://www.ncbi.nlm.nih.gov:80/entrez/query/static/clinical.html (accessed 16 July 2001).
13 User's guide to the medical literature *(JAMA)*. http://www.nzgg.org.nz/tools/resource_critical_appraisal.cfm#User Guides to Medical Literature (accessed 16 July 2001).
14 HSTAT Health Services/Technology Assessment Text. http://text.nlm.nih.gov/ (accessed 16 July 2001).
15 Fuller A, Wessel CB, Ginn DS, Martin TP. Quality filtering of the clinical literature by librarians and physicians. *Bull Med Libr Assoc* 1993;**81**(1):38–43.
16 Erickson S, Warner ER. The impact of individual tutorial sessions on MEDLINE use among obstetrics and gynaecology residents in an academic training programme: a randomized trial. *Med Educ* 1998;**32**(3):269–73.
17 Tsafrir J, Grinberg M. Who needs evidence-based health care? *Bull Med Libr Assoc* 1998;**86**(1):40–5.
18 Atlas M. The rise and fall of the medical mediated searcher. *Bull Med Libr Assoc* 2000;**88**(1):26–35.
19 Scherrer C, Dorsch JL. The evolving role of the librarian in evidence-based medicine. *Bull Med Libr Assoc* 1999;**87**(3):322–8.
20 Holtum E. Librarians, clinicians, evidence-based medicine, and the division of labour. *Bull Med Libr Assoc* 1999;**87**(4):404–7.

21 Obst O. Use of Internet resources by German medical professionals. *Bull Med Libr Assoc* 1998;**86**(4):528–33.

22 Curtis K, Weller AC, Hurd JM. Information-seeking behavior of health sciences faculty: the impact of new information technologies. *Bull Med Libr Assoc* 1997;**85**(4):402–10.

23 Cimpl K. Clinical medical librarianship: a review of the literature. *Bull Med Libr Assoc* 1985;**73**(1):21–8.

24 Schatz C, Whitehead SE. "Librarian for hire": contracting a librarian's services to external departments. *Bull Med Libr Assoc* 1995;**83**(4):469–72.

25 Wallingford K, Ruffin AB, Ginter KA, Spann ML, Johnson FE, Dutcher GA *et al.* Outreach activities of the National Library of Medicine: a five year review. *Bull Med Libr Assoc* 1996;**84**:116–21.

26 Rowlands JK, Forrester WH, McSean T. British Medical Association Library free MEDLINE service: survey of members taking part in an initial pilot project. *Bull Med Libr Assoc* 1996;**84**:116–21.

27 Humphreys BL, Ruffin AB, Cahn MA, Rambo N. Powerful connections for public health: the National Library of Medicine and the National Network of Libraries of Medicine. *Am J Public Health* 1999;**89**(11):1633–6.

28 PRISE. http://wwwlib.jr2.ox.ac.uk/prise/ (accessed 16 July 2001).

29 Vanderbilt University Medical Center. Eskind Biomedical Library Clinical Informatics Consult Service; [2 screens]. http://www.mc.vanderbilt.edu/biolib/services/cics.html (accessed 16 July 2001).

30 Klein M, Ross F. End-user searching: impetus for an expanding information management and technology role for the hospital librarian. *Bull Med Libr Assoc* 1997;**85**(3):260–8.

31 McGowan J, Winstead-Fry P. Problem Knowledge Couplers: reengineering evidence-based medicine through interdisciplinary development, decision support, and research. *Bull Med Libr Assoc* 1999;**87**(4):462–70.

32 Quintana Y. Intelligent medical information filtering. *Int J Med Inf* 1998;**51**(2–3):197–204.

33 Humphreys BL. Electronic health record meets digital library: a new environment for achieving an old goal. *J Am Med Inform Assoc* 2000;**7**(5):444–52.

34 Fuller S, Ketchell DS, Tarczy-Hornoch P, Masuda D. Integrating knowledge resources at the point of care: opportunities for librarians. *Bull Med Libr Assoc* 1999;**87**(4):393–407.

35 Guise N, Huber JT, Kafantaris SR, Guise D, Miller D, Giles DE Jr, *et al.* Preparing librarians to meet the challenges of today's health care environment. *J Am Med Inform Assoc* 1997;**4**(1):57–67.

36 Task Force Pro Libra. *Skills for the Knowledge Management: building a knowledge economy.* London: Task Force Pro Libra, 1999.

37 Palmer J, Streatfield D. Good diagnosis for the 21st century. *Library Association Record* 1995;**97**:153–4.

38 South Thames Research Application Programme. Critical Appraisal Skills (CAS)/ Finding Information in Networks and Databases (FIND) Training Project. http://www.netcomuk.co.uk/~strap/ (accessed 16 July 2001).

39 McKibbon A, Eady A, Marks S. *Evidence-based principles and practice.* Hamilton, Ontario: B.C. Decker Inc, 1999.

40 Marshall J. The impact of the hospital library on clinical decision-making: the Rochester study. *Bull Med Libr Assoc* 1992;**80**:169–78.

41 Klein M, Ross FV, Adams DL, Gilbert CM. Effects of on-line literature searching on length of stay and patient care costs. *Acad Med* 1994;**69**(6):489–95.

42 National Guideline Clearinghouse. Agency for Healthcare Research and Quality. http://www.guideline.gov/ (accessed 16 July 2001).

43 *Appraisal of NHS guidelines.* St. George's Hospital Medical School. Health Care Evaluation Unit. http://www.sghms.ac.uk/depts/phs/hceu/nhsguide.htm (accessed 16 July 2001).

44 Midwives Information and Resource Service. *Informed choice [leaflets].* Bristol: Midwives Information and Resource Service, 1995.

45 Oliver S, Rajan L, Turner H, Oakley A. *A pilot study of "Informed Choice" leaflets on positions in labour and routine ultrasound.* CRD report 7. York: University of York, NHS Centre for Reviews and Dissemination, 1996.

46 Cochrane Efficient Practice and Organisation of Care (EPOC). University of Aberdeen, Health Services Research Unit. http://www.abdn.ac.uk/public_health/hsru/epp/epoc.hti (accessed 16 July 2001).

47 Evans D, Haines A. *Implementing evidence-based changes in healthcare.* Abingdon: Radcliffe Medical Press, 2000.

48 Eve R, Golton I, Hodgkin P, Munro J, Musson G. *Learning from FACTS. Lessons from the Framework for Appropriate Care Throughout Sheffield (facts) project.* ScHARR Occasional paper no. 97/3. Sheffield: University of Sheffield, School of Health and Related Research, 1997.

49 NHS Centre for Reviews and Dissemination. Getting evidence into practice. *Effective HealthCare* 1999;5(1):1–16; http://www.york.ac.uk//crd/ehc5/warn.htm

4 Changing provider behaviour: an overview of systematic reviews of interventions to promote implementation of research findings by healthcare professionals

JEREMY GRIMSHAW, LIZ SHIRRAN, RUTH THOMAS, GRAHAM MOWATT, CYNTHIA FRASER, LISA BERO, ROBERTO GRILLI, EMMA HARVEY, ANDY OXMAN, AND MARY ANN O'BRIEN

> **Key messages**
> - Passive dissemination approaches are generally ineffective and unlikely to result in behaviour change when used alone.
> - Most other interventions are effective under some circumstances, none is effective under all circumstances.
> - Strategies that are generally effective include educational outreach (for prescribing behaviour) and reminders.
> - Multifaceted interventions based on assessment of potential barriers to change are more likely to be effective than single interventions.

There is increasing recognition of the failure to translate research findings into practice.[1] This has led to greater awareness of the importance of using active dissemination and implementation strategies. Whilst there is a substantial body of primary research evidence about the effectiveness of different strategies, this is widely dispersed across the medical literature and is not easily accessible to policy makers and professionals who make decisions about educational and quality improvement activities. This is analogous to the problems of identifying and retrieving evidence about the effectiveness of clinical interventions,[2] which has led to the recommendation that clinicians should use systematic reviews to solve clinical problems.[3] Fortunately, there are a growing number of systematic reviews of professional behaviour change interventions, which can inform policy decisions. However these reviews are published in a variety of sources that may not be easily accessible to policy makers. The aim of this overview was to use systematic methods to identify, appraise and summarise systematic reviews of professional educational or quality assurance interventions to improve quality of care. It updates a previous overview, which identified 18 systematic reviews published between 1966 and 1995.[4]

Methods

A full description of the methods (including search strategy used) has been published previously.[5,6] Briefly, reviews were included if they reported explicit selection criteria, concerned educational or quality assurance interventions targeted at health care professionals (qualified or undergoing postgraduate/professional training) and reported measures of professional performance and/or patient outcomes. We searched MEDLINE (between 1966 and July 1998), Healthstar (between 1975 and 1998) and the Cochrane Library (Issue 4 1998).[7] The list of potentially relevant systematic reviews was then circulated electronically to the Cochrane Effective Practice and Organisation of Care Group's list server; subscribers were asked to identify any potentially relevant published reviews that had been omitted. Two reviewers independently assessed reviews against the inclusion criteria. We identified seven reviews that were considered to be updates of previous reviews. For example, the Effective Health Care Bulletin on implementing clinical guidelines superseded the previous review by Grimshaw and Russell.[8,9] In these circumstances, we only abstracted data from the most recent update of a review. Two reviewers independently assessed the quality of included reviews and extracted data about the focus, inclusion criteria, main results and conclusions of the review. A previously validated checklist was used to assess quality.[10,11]

Results

We identified 41 systematic reviews that fulfilled our inclusion criteria covering a wide range of targeted behaviours and interventions. The reviews were of variable quality, with a median summary quality score of 4, indicating that they had some methodological flaws. Fifteen reviews focused on *broad strategies* (involving a variety of strategies across different targeted behaviours) including: continuing medical education (CME)[12-16], dissemination and implementation of guidelines;[8,17-22] programmes to enhance the quality and economy of primary care[23] and interventions to improve doctor-nurse collaboration.[24] Fourteen reviews focused on interventions targeting specific behaviours including: preventive care[25-30]; prescribing[31-33]; referrals[34]; test ordering[35]; and care at the end of life.[36] Fifteen reviews focused on the effectiveness of *specific interventions* (often across a range of different behaviours) including: printed educational materials[37]; outreach visits[38]; opinion leaders[39]; audit and feedback[40-44]; reminders and computerised decision support[41,45-47]; computer systems more generally[48,49]; feedback of cost data[50]; mass media[51]; and continuing quality improvement (CQI).[52] The reviews of specific interventions were categorised according to the EPOC taxonomy of interventions (see Box 4.1).[4]

Systematic reviews of broad strategies (see Appendix 4.1)

Reviews of CME

Davis and colleagues undertook a series of reviews of CME; the latest of which was published in 1995.[16] They identified 99 studies involving 160 comparisons of CME interventions. Improvements in at least 1 major endpoint were identified in 66% of comparisons. Single interventions likely to be effective included educational outreach, opinion leaders, patient mediated interventions and reminders. Multifaceted interventions and studies which undertook a 'gap analysis' to inform the development of the intervention were more likely to be successful.

Reviews of the introduction of clinical guidelines

Lomas undertook a review of passive dissemination of consensus recommendations and concluded that there was little evidence that passive dissemination alone resulted in provider behaviour change.[17] Grilli and Lomas undertook a review of factors influencing compliance with guideline recommendations; they found that compliance was lower for recommendations that were more complex and less trialable (i.e. recommendations that cannot be tried out and discarded easily).[18] An Effective Health Care Bulletin reviewed studies evaluating the introduction of guidelines; 81 out of 87 studies reported improvements with recommendations of guidelines and 12 out of 17 studies observed improvements in patient outcome.[8] It concluded that guidelines can change clinical practice and that guidelines were more likely to be effective if they took account of local circumstances, were disseminated by active educational interventions and were implemented by patient-specific reminders. There was inconclusive evidence about whether guidelines

31

Box 4.1   Interventions to promote professional behavioural change that could be used to implement research findings

- **Educational materials** – Distribution of published or printed recommendations for clinical care, including clinical practice guidelines, audio-visual materials and electronic publications. The materials may have been delivered personally or through personal or mass mailings.
- **Conferences** – Participation of health care providers in conferences, lectures, workshops or traineeships.
- **Local consensus process** – Inclusion of participating providers in discussion to ensure that they agree that the chosen clinical problem is important and the approach to managing the problem (i.e. the clinical practice guideline or definition of adequate care) is appropriate. The consensus process might also address the design of an intervention to improve performance.
- **Educational outreach visits** – Use of a trained person who meets with providers in their practice settings to provide information with the intent of changing the provider's performance. The information given may include feedback on the provider's performance.
- **Local opinion leaders** – Use of providers nominated by their colleagues as 'educationally influential'. The investigators must explicitly state that 'the opinion leaders were identified by their colleagues'.
- **Patient mediated interventions** – Any intervention aimed at changing the performance of health care providers where specific information was sought from or given to patients, for example direct mailings to patients; patient counselling delivered by someone other than the targeted providers; clinical information collected from patients by others and given to the provider; educational materials given to patients or placed in waiting rooms.
- **Audit and feedback** – Any summary of clinical performance over a specified period of time. Summarised information may include the average number of diagnostic tests ordered, the average cost per test or per patient, the average number of prescriptions written, the proportion of times a desired clinical action was taken, etc. The summary may also include recommendations for clinical care. The information may be given in a written or verbal format.
- **Reminders (manual or computerised)** – Any intervention that prompts the health care provider to perform a specific clinical action.
- **Marketing** – Use of personal interviewing, group discussion ('focus groups'), or a survey of targeted providers to identify barriers to change and the subsequent design of an intervention that addresses these barriers.
- **Multifaceted interventions** – Any intervention that includes two or more of the above.

developed by the end users (for example, local guidelines) were more likely to be effective than guidelines developed without involvement of the end users (for example, national guidelines). Oxman and colleagues undertook a review of 102 studies of interventions to improve the delivery of health care services.[19] They observed that dissemination activities resulted in little or no change in behaviour and that more complex interventions, whilst frequently effective, usually produced only moderate effects. They concluded that there were "no magic bullets" for provider behaviour change; there was a range of interventions that could lead to provider behaviour change but no single intervention was always effective for changing behaviour. Wensing and colleagues undertook a review of the effectiveness of introducing guidelines in primary care settings; they identified 61 studies which showed considerable variation in the effectiveness of a range of interventions.[22] Multifaceted interventions combining more than one intervention tended to be more effective but might be more expensive.

Other reviews of broad strategies

Yano and colleagues reviewed the effectiveness of programmes to improve specific aspects of primary care (for example, provision of preventive services, continuity of care)[23]; they identified a number of successful programmes but noted that there remain "significant gaps in our knowledge of how to improve aspects of care". For example, computer reminders and social influence interventions promoted preventive care. However, they found few studies evaluating interventions to improve primary care goals such as access to care, continuity of care, comprehensiveness of care, humanistic process, physical environment, aspects of patient outcome, shift in care from inpatient to outpatient settings. Zwarenstein and colleagues undertook a review of interventions to improve doctor–nurse collaboration[24]; despite the importance of multidisciplinary working in health care, they found no studies addressing this issue.

Systematic reviews of interventions to improve specific behaviours (see Appendix 4.2)

Interventions to improve preventive care

Two reviews undertook broad reviews of a range of interventions to influence all aspects of prevention. Lomas and Haynes reviewed 32 studies; 28 out of 31 studies reported significant improvements in process of care and 4 out of 13 studies reported significant findings in patient outcomes.[25] Hulscher reviewed 58 studies of interventions to improve preventive care in primary care settings[29]; she identified a range of effective interventions and concluded that multifaceted interventions including reminders are effective, but noted that such interventions might incur greater cost. Gyorkos and colleagues reviewed interventions to improve immunisation; interventions aimed at hospitalised patients were most effective for influenza immunisations, client and system oriented interventions were effective for pneumococcal immunisations and system oriented interventions were effective for measles, mumps and rubella (MMR) immunisations.[26] Mandelblatt and Kanetsky reviewed interventions to improve mammography and found reminder systems and audit and feedback were generally effective.[27] Snell reviewed interventions to increase screening rates for breast, cervical and colorectal cancer.[28] Patient-directed and provider-directed interventions were both effective; however, interventions which targeted both professionals and patients were less successful. The effectiveness of patient-directed interventions decreased with the number of interventions employed, whereas the effectiveness of provider-directed interventions increased when up to three interventions were employed. It was not possible to identify which patient-directed interventions were more likely to be successful. Provider-directed interventions which were multifaceted and included targeted awareness and behaviour cues appeared optimal. Lancaster and colleagues reviewed the effectiveness of training professionals about smoking cessation; they found that such training had only a modest effect on smoking cessation rates; there was one extra quitter for about every 50 patients advised by a trained rather than an untrained physician.[30]

Interventions to improve prescribing

Soumerai and colleagues reviewed interventions to improve prescribing.[31] They found that mailed educational materials alone were generally ineffective, educational outreach approaches and ongoing feedback were generally effective and there was insufficient evidence to determine the effectiveness of reminder systems and group education. They also observed that poorly controlled studies were more likely to report significant results compared to adequately controlled studies, emphasising the need for rigorous evaluations of dissemination and implementation strategies. Anderson and colleagues updated this review and found that feedback including specific recommendations for change in the use of medications was more likely to change behaviour than feedback providing a description of current behaviour.[33]

Interventions to improve other behaviours

Grimshaw undertook a review of interventions to improve outpatient referrals[34]; only four studies were identified that showed mixed effects and concluded that it was difficult to draw any firm conclusions on the basis of the review. Solomon and colleagues reviewed 49 studies of interventions to modify test ordering behaviour[35]; 15 out of 21 studies targeting a single behavioural factor were successful, whereas 24 out of 28 studies targeting more than one behavioural factor were successful. They concluded that the majority of interventions were successful and that there was a trend towards greater success with multifaceted interventions.

Systematic reviews of specific interventions (see Appendix 4.3)

Dissemination of educational materials

Freemantle and colleagues reviewed 11 studies evaluating the effects of the dissemination of educational materials (see Box 4.1).[37] None of the studies found statistically significant improvements in practice.

Educational outreach visits

Thomson and colleagues reviewed the effectiveness of educational outreach visits (see Box 4.1).[38] They identified 18 studies mainly targeting prescribing behaviour. The majority of studies observed statistical improvements in care (especially when social marketing techniques were used)[53] although the effects were small to moderate. Educational outreach was observed to be more effective than audit and feedback in one study. The cost effectiveness of educational outreach was unclear.

Local opinion leaders

Thomson and colleagues reviewed the effectiveness of local opinion leaders (see Box 4.1).[39] They identified six studies; five out of six trials observed improvements in at least one process of care variable although these results were only statistically and clinically important in one trial. One of three trials observed an improvement in patient outcome that was of practical importance. Local opinion leaders were observed to be more effective than group audit and feedback in one study. They concluded that using local opinion leaders resulted in mixed effects and that further research was required before the widespread use of this intervention could be justified.

Audit and feedback

Buntinx and colleagues found that feedback was less effective than reminders for reducing the utilisation of diagnostic tests.[41] Balas and colleagues reviewed 12 evaluations of physician profiling defined as "peer-comparison feedback"[42]; 10 studies observed statistically significant improvements, however the effects were small. They concluded that peer comparison alone is unlikely to result in substantial quality improvement or cost-control and may be inefficient. Thomson and colleagues undertook a review of audit and feedback (see Box 4.1).[43,44] They identified 13 studies which compared audit and feedback to a no intervention control group, eight reported statistically significant changes in favour of the experimental group in at least one major outcome measure, however the effects were small to moderate. The review concluded that "audit and feedback can be effective in improving performance, in particular for prescribing and test ordering, although the effects are small to moderate" and that the "widespread use of audit and feedback" was not supported by the review.

Reminders (manual or computerised)

Hunt and colleagues reviewed the effectiveness of computer based decision support systems (CDSS).[47] Significant improvements were observed in: 9 of 15 drug dosing studies; 1 of 5 studies on diagnosis; 14 of 19 studies on prevention; 19 of 26 studies on general management of a problem; and 4 of 7 studies on patient outcome. They concluded that CDSS might enhance clinical performance for most aspects of care, but not diagnosis.

Other interventions

There were two broader reviews on the effects of computerised systems. Sullivan and Mitchell reviewed 30 studies on the effects of computers on primary care consultations[48]; they observed that immunisation, other preventive tasks and other aspects of performance improved, however consultation time lengthened and there was a reduction in patient-initiated social contact. Balas and colleagues reviewed 98 trials of computerised information systems.[49] They found that different information interventions improved care, including: provider prompts; patient prompts; computer assisted patient education and computer assisted treatment planners. Beilby reviewed six studies on the effects of feedback on cost information to general practitioners[50]; five out of the six studies observed significant improvements. Grilli and colleagues reviewed 17 studies of the effects of mass media interventions on health services utilisation[51]; seven studies observed statistical improvements (following re-analysis), meta-analysis suggested that mass media campaigns had an effect on health services utilisation. Shortell and colleagues undertook a systematic review of CQI programmes.[52] They identified 43 single site studies (41 used an uncontrolled before and after design) and 13 multi-site (12 of which used a cross sectional or uncontrolled before and after design); the results from the uncontrolled before and after or cross sectional studies suggested that CQI was effective, whereas all randomised studies observed no effect. They concluded that the predominance of single site study designs made it difficult to attribute the observed effects to CQI.

Discussion

These systematic reviews identified a variety of dissemination and implementation strategies that are effective under certain conditions, although none are effective under all circumstances.[19] Passive dissemination (for example, mailing educational materials to targeted clinicians) is generally ineffective and is unlikely to result in behaviour change when used alone; however this approach may be useful for raising awareness of the desired behaviour change. Active approaches are more likely to be effective but also likely to be more costly. Interventions of variable effectiveness include audit and feedback and use of local opinion leaders. Generally effective strategies include educational outreach (for prescribing behaviour) and reminders. Multifaceted interventions based on assessment of potential barriers to change are more likely to be effective than single interventions.

Systematic reviews of rigorous evaluations provide the best evidence about the effectiveness of different provider behaviour change strategies. Whilst the current evidence base is incomplete, it provides valuable insights into the likely effectiveness of different interventions. Future quality improvement or educational activities should be informed by the findings of such systematic reviews.

Acknowledgements

A full report of this overview was published in Medical Care[5] and a summary of this overview was published as part of an Effective Health Care Bulletin.[6] The Health Services Research Unit is funded by the Chief Scientist Office, Scottish Executive Department of Health. The Cochrane Effective Practice and Organisation of Care Group is funded by the Department of Health, United Kingdom. This work was partly funded by the NHS Centre for Reviews and Dissemination, United Kingdom. The views expressed are those of the authors and not the funding bodies. Nick Freemantle contributed to the original overview.

References

1 Grol R, Grimshaw JM. Evidence-based implementation of evidence-based medicine. *Jt Comm J Qual Improv* 1999;**25**:503–13.
2 Haynes RB, Sackett DL, Tugwell P. Problems in handling of clinical research evidence by medical practitioners. *Arch Intern Med* 1983;**143**:1971–5.
3 Guyatt G, Rennie D. Users' guides to the medical literature. *JAMA* 1993;**270**:2096–7.
4 Bero LA, Grilli R, Grimshaw JM, Harvey E, Oxman AD, Thomson MA. Closing the gap between research and practice: an overview of systematic reviews of interventions to promote the implementation of research findings. *BMJ* 1998;**317**:265–8.

5 Grimshaw JM, Shirran L, Thomas RE, Mowatt G, Fraser C, Bero L *et al.* Changing provider behaviour: an overview of systematic reviews of interventions. *Medical Care* 2001 (*in press*).

6 NHS Centre for Reviews and Dissemination. Getting evidence into practice. *Effective Health Care* 1999;5(1):1–16. (Also available from: http://www.york.ac.uk/inst/crd/ehc51.pdf.)

7 The Cochrane Library, Issue 4, 1998. Oxford: Update Software. Updated quarterly.

8 Effective Health Care. Implementing clinical guidelines. Can guidelines be used to improve clinical practice? *Effective Health Care* 1994;1(8).

9 Grimshaw JM, Russell IT. Effect of clinical guidelines on medical practice. A systematic review of rigorous evaluations. *Lancet* 1993;342:1317–22.

10 Oxman AD, Guyatt GH. The science of reviewing research. *Ann N Y Acad Sci* 1993;703:123–31.

11 Oxman AD. Checklists for review articles. *BMJ* 1994;309:648–51.

12 Bertram DA, Brooks-Bertram PA. The evaluation of continuing medical education: a literature review. *Health Educ Monogr* 1977;5(4):330–62.

13 Lloyd JS, Abrahamson S. Effectiveness of continuing medical education: a review of the evidence. *Eval Health Prof* 1979;2(3):251–80.

14 Beaudry JS. The effectiveness of continuing medical education: a quantitative synthesis. *J Cont Educ Health Prof* 1989;9:285–307.

15 Waddell DL. The effects of continuing education on nursing practice: a meta-analysis. *J Contin Educ Nurs* 1991;22:113–18.

16 Davis DA, Thomson MA, Oxman AD, Haynes RB. Changing physician performance: a systematic review of the effect of continuing medical education strategies. *JAMA* 1995;274:700–5.

17 Lomas J. Words without action? The production, dissemination, and impact of consensus recommendations. *Annu Rev Public Health* 1991;12:41–65.

18 Grilli R, Lomas J. Evaluating the message: the relationship between compliance rate and the subject of a practice guideline. *Med Care* 1994;32:202–13.

19 Oxman AD, Thomson MA, Davis DA, Haynes RB. No magic bullets: a systematic review of 102 trials of interventions to improve professional practice. *CMAJ* 1995;153:1423–31.

20 Davis DA, Taylor-Vaisey A. Translating guidelines into practice. A systematic review of theoretical concepts, practical experience and research evidence in the adoption of clinical practice guidelines. *CMAJ* 1997;157:408–16.

21 Worrall G, Chaulk P, Freake D. The effects of clinical practice guidelines on patient outcomes in primary care: a systematic review. *CMAJ* 1997;156:1705–12.

22 Wensing M, van der Weijden T, Grol R. Implementing guidelines and innovations in general practice: which interventions are effective? *Br J Gen Pract* 1998;48:991–7.

23 Yano EM, Fink A, Hirsch SH, Robbins AS, Rubenstein LV. Helping practices reach primary care goals. Lessons from the literature. *Arch Intern Med* 1995;155:1146–56.

24 Zwarenstein M, Bryant W, Bailie R, Sibthorpe B. Interventions to change collaboration between nurses and doctors (Cochrane Review). In: *The Cochrane Library*. Oxford: Update Software, Issue 42, 1997.

25 Lomas J, Haynes RB. A taxonomy and critical review of tested strategies of the application of clinical practice recommendations: from "official" to "individual" clinical policy. *Am J Prev Med.* 1988;2:77–94.

26 Gyorkos TW, Tannenbaum TN, Abrahamowicz M, Bedard L, Carsley J, Fanco ED *et al.* Evaluation of the effectiveness of immunisation delivery methods. *Can J Public Health* 1994;85(Suppl 1):S14–30.

27 Mandelblatt J, Kanetsky PA. Effectiveness of interventions to enhance physician screening for breast cancer. *J Fam Pract* 1995;40:162–71.

28 Snell JL, Buck EL. Increasing cancer screening: a meta-analysis. *Prev Med* 1996;25:702–7.

29 Hulscher M. *Implementing prevention in general practice: a study on cardiovascular disease.* PhD thesis. Nijmegen: University of Nijmegen, 1998.

30 Lancaster T, Silagy C, Gray S, Fowler G. The effectiveness of training health professionals to provide smoking cessation interventions: systematic review of randomised controlled trials (Cochrane Review). In: *The Cochrane Library*. Oxford: Update Software, Issue 4, 1998.

31 Soumerai SB, McLaughlin TJ, Avorn J. Improving drug prescribing in primary care: a critical analysis of the experimental literature. *Milbank Q* 1989;**67**:268–317.
32 Gurwitz JH, Soumerai SB, Avorn J. Improving medication prescribing and utilisation in the nursing home. *J Am Geriatr Soc* 1990;**38**:542–52.
33 Anderson GM, Lexchin J. Strategies for improving prescribing practice. *CMAJ* 1996;**154**:1013–17.
34 Grimshaw JM. *Evaluation of four quality assurance initiatives to improve out-patient referrals from general practice to hospital.* PhD Thesis. Aberdeen: University of Aberdeen, 1998.
35 Solomon DH, Hashimoto H, Daltroy L, Liang MH. Techniques to improve physicians' uses of diagnostic tests. *JAMA* 1998;**280**:2020–7.
36 Hanson LC, Tulsky JA, Danis M. Can clinical interventions change care at the end of life? *Ann Intern Med* 1997;**126**:381–8.
37 Freemantle N, Harvey EL, Wolf F, Grimshaw JM, Grilli R, Bero LA. Printed educational materials to improve the behaviour of health care professionals and patient outcomes (Cochrane Review). In: *The Cochrane Library.* Oxford: Update Software, Issue 3, 1996.
38 Thomson MA, Oxman AD, Davis DA, Haynes RB, Freemantle N, Harvey EL. Outreach visits to improve health professional practice and health care outcomes (Cochrane Review). In: *The Cochrane Library.* Oxford: Update Software, Issue 4, 1997.
39 Thomson MA, Oxman AD, Davis DA, Haynes RB, Freemantle N, Harvey EL. Local opinion leaders to improve health professional practice and health care outcomes (Cochrane Review). In: *The Cochrane Library.* Oxford: Update Software, Issue 3, 1997.
40 Mugford M, Banfield P, O'Hanlon M. Effects of feedback of information on clinical practice: a review. *BMJ* 1991;**303**:398–402.
41 Buntinx F, Winkens R, Grol R, Knottnerus JA. Influencing diagnostic and preventative performance in ambulatory care by feedback and reminders. A Review. *Fam Pract* 1993;**10**:219–28.
42 Balas EA, Boren SA, Brown GD, Ewigman BG, Mitchell JA, Perkoff GT. Effect of physician profiling on utilisation. *J Gen Intern Med* 1996;**11**:584–90.
43 Thomson MA, Oxman AD, Davis DA, Haynes RB, Freemantle N, Harvey EL. Audit and feedback to improve health professional practice and health care outcomes Part I (Cochrane Review). In: *The Cochrane Library.* Oxford: Update Software, Issue 1, 1998.
44 Thomson MA, Oxman AD, Davis DA, Haynes RB, Freemantle N, Harvey EL. Audit and feedback to improve health professional practice and health care outcomes Part II (Cochrane Review). In: *The Cochrane Library.* Oxford: Update Software, Issue 1, 1998.
45 Austin SM, Balas EA, Mitchell JA, Ewigman GB. Effect of physician reminders on preventative care: meta-analysis of randomized clinical trials. *Proc Annu Symp Comput Appl Med Care* 1994;121–4.
46 Shea S, DuMouchel W, Bahamonde L. A meta-analysis of 16 randomized controlled trials to evaluate computer-based clinical reminder systems for preventative care in the ambulatory setting. *J Am Med Inform Assoc* 1996;**3**:399–409.
47 Hunt DL, Haynes RB, Hanna SE, Smith K. Effects of computer-based clinical decision support systems on physician performance and patient outcomes. A systematic review. *JAMA* 1998;**280**:1339–46.
48 Sullivan F, Mitchell E. Has general practitioner computing made a difference to patient care? A systematic review of published reports. *BMJ* 1995;**311**:848–52.
49 Balas EA, Austin SM, Mitchell J, Ewigman BG, Bopp KD, Brown GD. The clinical value of computerised information services. *Arch Fam Med* 1996;**5**:271–78.
50 Beilby J, Silagy CA. Trials of providing costing information to general practitioners: a systematic review. *MJA* 1997;**167**:89–92.
51 Grilli R, Freemantle N, Minozzi S, Domenighetti G, Finer D. Impact of mass media on health services utilisation (Cochrane Review). In: *The Cochrane Library.* Oxford: Update Software, Issue 3, 1998.
52 Shortell SM, Bennett CL, Byck GR. Assessing the impact of continuous quality improvement on clinical practice: what it will take to accelerate progress. *Milbank Q* 1998;**76**:1–37.
53 Soumerai SB, Avorn J. Principles of educational outreach ('academic detailing') to improve clinical decision making. *JAMA* 1990;**263**:549–56.

Appendix 4.1 Summary of systematic reviews of the effects of broadly defined implementation strategies on professional practice

Key: RCT = Randomised controlled trial
            CCT = Controlled clinical trial
            CA   = Controlled after
            UA   = Uncontrolled after
            BA   = Before/after
            CBA = Controlled before/after
            XS   = Cross sectional
            ITS   = Interrupted time series

Continuing medical education strategies

Bertram 1977[12] *Effectiveness of continuing medical education (CME)*

Inclusion criteria:

- Study designs: Any study design
- Participants: Practising physicians
- Intervention: Any evaluation
- Outcomes: Not explicitly stated
- Period: Not explicitly stated
- Other: Only English language studies included

Main results

- 65 studies met the inclusion criteria.
- 4 of 10 studies targeting physician behaviour reported improvements.
- 4 studies targeting patient health status had unclear results.
- Statistical significance of findings unclear.

Authors' main conclusions

- Cannot make firm conclusions regarding the effectiveness of CME. Generalisation hindered by inadequate evaluation of methods, insufficient programme description, lack of defining terms and incomparability among the CME programmes.
- Need for further research to adequately investigate the importance of physician behaviour and patient health status.

Lloyd 1979[13] *Effectiveness of continuing medical education (CME)*

Inclusion criteria:

- Study designs: Not explicitly stated (included CA, RCT, CBA, BA, XS)
- Participants: Physicians who have completed undergraduate and graduate medical education

- Intervention: Continuing medical education interventions
- Outcomes: Physician competence (knowledge, attitudes), physician performance and patient health status
- Period: 1960–1977

Main results

- 47 studies met the inclusion criteria.
- 13 of 22 assessing competence observed improvements: 10 of these 13 reported significant improvements (including 1 of 2 RCT and 2 of 4 CBA).
- 11 of 26 studies assessing performance observed significant improvements (including 2 of 2 RCT and 2 of 6 CBA).
- 4 of 4 assessing patient health status observed improvements: 2 reported significant improvements (including 1 of 1 RCT).

Authors' main conclusions

- About half of the studies reported demonstrable improvements in competence, performance or patient health status.
- Methodological shortcomings of studies make it impossible to conclude that the improvements were caused by CME.
- Further research and development of CME is required.
- The definition of CME should be broadened to include interventions to change provider performance.

Beaudry 1989[14] *Effectiveness of CME*

Inclusion criteria:

- Study designs: RCT, CBA
- Participants: Not explicitly stated (physicians)
- Intervention: Continuing medical education interventions
- Outcomes: Physician knowledge and performance, patient health status
- Period: 1931–1986

Main results

- 63 studies met the inclusion criteria.
- 41 studies reported sufficient data to calculate effect sizes for 282 outcomes.
- CME showed a 'strong' effect on knowledge (standardised mean difference (SMD) 0·79) and a 'moderate' (not statistically significant) effect on performance (SMD 0·55) and health status (SMD 0·37).

Authors' main conclusions

- There are important inadequacies in the design and reporting of evaluations of CME programs and cross-study comparisons are

41

difficult, limiting conclusions about the impact of specific characteristics of CME.

- These results must be interpreted cautiously and do not imply any normative standards for overall program performance.

Waddell 1991[15] *Effectiveness of continuing education on nursing practice (CME)*

Inclusion criteria:

- Study designs: Not explicitly stated (unable to determine designs included)
- Participants: Not explicitly stated (nurses)
- Intervention: Continuing nursing education interventions
- Outcomes: Practice-related behaviours
- Period: Not explicitly stated

Main results

- 34 studies met the inclusion criteria.
- Education positively affects nursing practice. The average member of an intervention group performed as well as, or better than, 77% of the members of control groups.
- Findings that related to mediating effects were inconclusive.

Authors' main conclusions

- The overall effect size supports the hypothesis that continuing education positively affects nursing practice.
- There was a greater likelihood of effect when learners were from the same practice environment and planned their continuing education activities accordingly.

Davis 1995[16] *Effectiveness of continuing medical education (CME)*

Inclusion criteria:

- Study designs: RCT, CCT
- Participants: Health professionals
- Intervention: Educational intervention directed at changing clinical behaviour or health outcomes
- Outcomes: Objective measurement of physician performance or health care outcomes
- Period: 1975–1994

Main results

- 99 studies met the inclusion criteria comprising 160 comparisons.
- Improvements in at least one major endpoint in physician

42

performance or patient outcome of care were identified in 66% of comparisons.

- Single strategies likely to be effective included educational outreach, opinion leaders, patient mediated interventions and reminders. Multifaceted interventions were more likely to be successful.
- Studies which undertook a gap analysis or needs analysis to inform the development of the interventions appeared more likely to be positive.

Authors' main conclusions

- Widely used CME delivery methods such as conferences have little direct impact on improving professional practice.
- CME providers seldom use more effective methods such as systematic practice-based interventions and outreach visits.

Introduction of clinical guidelines

Lomas 1991[17] *Impact of dissemination of consensus recommendations*

Inclusion criteria:

- Study designs: Not explicitly stated (included ITS, BA, XS studies)
- Participants: Physicians
- Intervention: Dissemination of consensus recommendations
- Outcomes: Physician behaviour or percent conformity with consensus recommendations
- Period: 1980–1991

Main results

- 19 studies met the inclusion criteria.
- 6 of 10 that used actual practice data found no impact, 2 found minor impact and 2 found major impact. Only one study using self-report showed a major impact.
- Statistical significance of findings unclear.

Authors' main conclusions

- Existing evaluations have found little or no evidence that dissemination of consensus recommendations alone lead to action.

Grilli 1994[18] *Relationship between compliance rates and the subject of practice guidelines*

Inclusion criteria:

- Study designs: Not explicitly stated (CBA, XS included)
- Participants: Providers

43

- Intervention: Not explicitly stated (publication or dissemination of guidelines developed by official organisations)
- Outcomes: Compliance rates with guidelines
- Period: 1980–1991
- Other: Studies of locally developed guidelines and trials of implementation strategies were excluded. Only English language studies included

Main results

- 23 studies with 143 recommendations addressing 70 different aspects of medical practice met the inclusion criteria.
- The overall mean compliance rate was 55%.
- High complexity recommendations had significantly lower compliance rates.
- Highly trialable recommendations had significantly higher compliance rates.
- There was no significant difference in compliance between recommendations with high versus low observability.

Authors' main conclusions

- There was a high degree of variation in reported compliance rates and a low average compliance rate.
- High complexity/low trialability recommendations may require more active dissemination activities to predispose practitioners to change their behaviour than low complexity/high trialability recommendations where efforts can focus more quickly on enabling change at the local level.

Effective Health Care 1994[8] *Effectiveness of strategies for implementing clinical practice guidelines*

Inclusion criteria:

- Study designs: RCT, CBA, ITS
- Participants: Medical staff
- Intervention: Guideline dissemination and/or implementation strategies
- Outcomes: Process of care or patient outcome
- Period: 1976–1994

Main results

- 91 studies met the inclusion criteria.
- 81 of 87 studies reported significant improvements in adherence to recommendations of practice guidelines.
- 12 of 17 that reported patient outcome also reported significant improvements.

Authors' main conclusions

- Properly developed guidelines can change clinical practice and may lead to changes in patient outcome.
- Guidelines are more likely to be effective if they take into account local circumstances, are disseminated by an active educational intervention, and implemented by patient specific reminders.

Oxman 1995[19] *Effectiveness of interventions to improve delivery of health care services*

Inclusion criteria:

- Study designs: RCT
- Participants: Health care providers
- Intervention: 10 interventions to improve delivery of health care services
- Outcomes: Objective assessment of provider performance or health outcome
- Period: 1970–1993

Main results

- 102 studies met the inclusion criteria.
- Disseminating-only strategies such as mailed, unsolicited materials or conferences used alone resulted in little or no change in behaviour.
- More complex interventions ranged from ineffective to highly effective, but effects were most often moderate.

Authors' main conclusions

- There are no magic bullets for improving the quality of health care, but there is a range of interventions available that, if used appropriately, can lead to important improvements in professional practice and patient outcomes.

Davis 1997[20] *Effectiveness of strategies for implementing clinical practice guidelines*

Inclusion criteria:

- Study designs: Not clear (RCT were '*emphasised*')
- Participants: Not explicitly stated (practising clinicians)
- Intervention: Guideline implementation strategies
- Outcomes: Not clear (studies with objective measures of provider behaviour or health status were '*emphasised*')
- Period: 1990–1996

Main results

- Unclear how many trials met the inclusion criteria.
- Weak interventions included didactic traditional CME and mailings; moderately effective interventions included audit and feedback; relatively strong interventions included reminder systems, academic detailing and multiple interventions.

Authors' main conclusions

- Future implementation strategies should be based upon an understanding of the forces and variables influencing practice and through the use of methods that are practice- and community-based rather than didactic.

Worrall 1997[21] *Effectiveness of introduction of clinical practice guidelines on patient outcomes in primary care*

Inclusion criteria:

- Study designs: RCT, CCT
- Participants: Primary care professionals
- Intervention: Guideline dissemination and/or implementation strategies
- Outcomes: Patient outcomes
- Period: 1980–1995

Main results

- 13 studies met the inclusion criteria.
- 5 studies observed statistically significant improvements in patient outcomes of care.

Authors' main conclusions

- There is little evidence that use of guidelines improves patient outcomes in primary medical care.
- Research is needed to determine whether the newer, evidence-based CPGs have an effect on patient outcomes.

Wensing 1998[22] *Effectiveness of interventions to implement guidelines or innovations in general practice*

Inclusion criteria:

- Study designs: RCT, CCT, CBA
- Participants: General practitioners
- Intervention: Any intervention to improve professional practice
- Outcomes: Provider behaviour
- Period: 1980–1994

Main results

- 61 studies met the inclusion criteria.
  ### Single interventions
- 8 of 17 studies of information transfer observed significant improvements.
- 14 of 15 studies of information linked to performance observed significant improvements.
- 3 of 5 studies of learning through social influence observed significant improvements.
- 3 of 3 studies of management support observed significant improvements.
  ### Multifaceted interventions
- 8 of 20 studies of information transfer with information linked to performance observed significant improvements.
- 7 of 8 studies of information transfer with learning through social influence observed significant improvements.
- 6 of 7 studies of information transfer with management support observed significant improvements.
- 3 of 3 studies of information linked to performance with learning through social influence observed significant improvements.
- 5 of 6 studies of use of more than 3 interventions observed significant improvements.

Authors' main conclusions

- Strategies combining more interventions may be more expensive but also more effective.
- All interventions show considerable variation in their effectiveness.
- The combination of information transfer and learning through social influence or management support can be effective and so can reminders or feedback.
- Need for more research to determine if other interventions are effective.

Other broadly defined interventions

Yano 1995[23] *Effectiveness of programmes to enhance quality and economy of primary care*

Inclusion criteria:

- Study designs: Not explicitly stated (included RCT and other unspecified designs)
- Participants: Primary care professionals, students, patients

- Intervention: Primary care programmes, defined as "a set of specific activities designed to address one or more primary care goals on a system or practice wide basis"
- Outcomes: 14 primary care goals
- Period: 1980–1992

Main results

- 36 studies were included from a total of 72 identified studies meeting the inclusion criteria.
- Programmes to improve preventive services, management/co-ordination of care, appropriate use of services and to reduce physician ordered services were largely successful.
- Programmes to improve patient outcome, access, efficiency, to decrease costs/charges and to shift care from inpatient to outpatient settings were sometimes successful.
- Programmes to improve continuity of care, comprehensiveness of care, technical aspects of care, humanistic process, physical environment were largely unsuccessful.

Authors' main conclusions

- Studies of successful programmes were identified although there are "significant gaps in our knowledge of how to improve aspects of care".
- Primary care practices can implement several programmes to improve prevention and access and to reduce costs and use of unnecessary services.

Zwarenstein 1997[24] *Effectiveness of interventions to improve nurse–doctor collaboration*

Inclusion criteria:

- Study designs: RCT, CBA, ITS
- Participants: Doctors and nurses in primary or secondary care
- Intervention: Interventions to improve collaboration between doctors and nurses sharing care of patients
- Outcomes: Objectively measured attitudes and behaviour or any direct effects upon patient care
- Period: Not explicitly stated (Medline search completed in 1996)

Main results

- No studies met the inclusion criteria.

Authors' main conclusions

- No reliable evidence of effect is available.

- Need to research the barriers to collaboration and the effectiveness of interventions designed to improve collaboration.
- The possibility of inadequate indexing in bibliographic databases acknowledged.

Appendix 4.2 Summary of systematic reviews of the effects of implementation strategies targeting specific behaviours

Key: RCT = Randomised controlled trial
CCT = Controlled clinical trial
CA   = Controlled after
UA   = Uncontrolled after
BA   = Before/after
CBA = Controlled before/after
XS   = Cross sectional
ITS = Interrupted time series

Interventions to improve preventive care

Lomas 1988[25] *Educational and administrative strategies to promote preventive care*

Inclusion criteria:

- Study designs: RCT
- Participants: Physicians in practice or training
- Intervention: Educational and administrative strategies to improve performance of physicians with (preventive care) recommendations
- Outcomes: Physician performance or patient outcome
- Period: 1975–1987

Main results

- 32 studies met the inclusion criteria.
- 28 of 31 observed significant improvements in practitioner performance.
- 4 of 13 studies observed significant improvements in patient outcomes.

Authors' main conclusions

- Many dissemination and application tactics in common use merit further rigorous testing or abandonment, particularly patient-centred strategies.

- Because of the complexity of the determinants of clinical practice, simple solutions are unlikely.
- Those who promulgate practice recommendations should ensure dissemination and application of their recommendations.

Gyorkos 1994[26] *Interventions to improve immunisation coverage*

Inclusion criteria:

- Study designs: Studies comparing one or more interventions with a control group (RCT, CCT, 'Cohort')
- Participants: Human population in developed countries
- Intervention: Delivery methods to improve immunisation
- Outcomes: "No restriction was placed on the type of outcome measure" (immunisation coverage)
- Period: 1979–1992
- Other: Only studies in French and English included

Main results

- 54 studies met the inclusion criteria.
- The largest improvements in influenza immunisation coverage resulted from interventions aimed at hospitalised patients.
- Both client- and system-oriented interventions targeted at high risk hospitalised patients can achieve high coverage rates for pneumococcal immunisation.
- One study reported on Hepatitis B immunisation coverage. The generalisability to other populations was very limited.
- Studies of system-oriented interventions reported larger improvements than studies of client-oriented interventions for MMR.

Authors' main conclusions

- Many factors affect improvements in immunisation coverage, including characteristics of the target populations, baseline coverage rate, vaccine efficacy, and the knowledge, attitudes and practice of local health care providers.
- Variation in these determinants limits the generalisability of results from individual studies.

Mandelblatt 1995[27] *Effectiveness of interventions to improve physician screening for breast cancer*

Inclusion criteria:

- Study designs: RCT, CCT
- Participants: Physicians
- Intervention: Interventions to enhance physician behaviours regarding breast cancer screening

- Outcomes: Not explicitly stated
- Period: 1980–1993
- Other: Only studies in USA considered

Main results

- 20 studies met the inclusion criteria.
- Successful interventions included reminder systems, audit and feedback.
- There was limited evidence that physician and patient education were successful in community based settings only.

Authors' main conclusions

- Physician based interventions can be effective in increasing screening use.

Snell 1996[28] *Effectiveness of interventions to increase screening rates for breast, cervical and colorectal cancer*

Inclusion criteria:

- Study designs: Not explicitly stated (unable to determine designs included)
- Participants: Physicians and patients in primary care
- Intervention: Interventions to increase cancer screening rates
- Outcomes: Not explicitly stated (appointments scheduled and kept, adherent patients)
- Period: 1989–1994

Main results

- 38 studies met the inclusion criteria.
- Effect size decreased as the number of interventions targeting patients increased.
- As the number of interventions increased so did the effect size when targeting physicians.
- A combination of during and outside visit interventions led to a greater effect size in physicians.

Authors' main conclusions

- Multifaceted approaches were more effective at changing physician behaviour. Need for further research to investigate this non-linear relationship.
- Not clear which patient focused interventions were most effective.
- Physician and patient interventions were equally successful, no added benefit of targeting both.
- Focused approaches were more effective than the shotgun approach.

Hulscher 1998[29] *Effectiveness of alternative interventions to improve the delivery of preventive care*

Inclusion criteria:

- Study designs: RCT, CBA, ITS
- Participants: Primary care professionals
- Intervention: Any professional, organisational, financial or regulatory intervention
- Outcomes: Objectively measured professional performance or patient outcomes
- Period: 1966–1995

Main results

- 58 studies met the inclusion criteria.

Single interventions

- 5 of 8 studies of education observed significant improvements.
- 1 of 3 studies of individual instruction observed significant improvements.
- 2 of 4 studies of feedback observed significant improvements.
- 9 of 13 studies of physician reminders observed significant improvements.
- A small difference was found to favour organisational interventions and no evidence of effect was found on the effect of financial or regulatory interventions.

Multifaceted interventions

- 9 of 23 studies of interventions including feedback observed significant improvements.
- 17 of 17 studies including physician reminders observed significant improvements.
- Other combinations produced mixed results.

Authors' main conclusions

- Effective interventions are available to increase preventive activities in primary care. Multifaceted interventions including reminders resulted in the greatest improvement in effectiveness but may incur greater cost.
- Need for further research to determine what elements of interventions work, why they work, and at what cost.

Lancaster 1998[30] *Effectiveness of interventions to improve the delivery of smoking cessation programs by health professionals*

Inclusion criteria:

- Study designs: RCT
- Participants: Healthcare professionals

- Intervention: Training interventions to provide smoking cessation interventions
- Outcomes: Process variables and rates of abstinence
- Period: Not explicitly stated

Main results

- 9 studies met the inclusion criteria.
- Training providers can significantly improve the odds of their patients quitting smoking (OR 1·48, 95% CI 1·20–1·83).
- The use of reminders in addition to training had a statistically significant effect in two studies (OR 2·37, 95% CI 1·43–3·92) and the addition of nicotine gum may also improve the impact of training.

Authors' main conclusions

- Educational strategies directed towards health care professionals to support them in helping patients to quit smoking appear to have only a measurable effect on quit rates.
- There was also a modest effect on patient outcome.

Interventions to improve prescribing

Soumerai 1989[31] *Improving drug prescribing in primary care*

Inclusion criteria:

- Study designs: RCT, CBA, ITS, BA, UA
- Participants: Physicians
- Intervention: Non regulatory, non commercial programs to improve drug prescribing
- Outcomes: Drug prescribing
- Period: 1970–1988
- Other: Non English language studies, reports of pure regulatory interventions and changes in financial incentives to patients were excluded

Main results

- 44 studies met the inclusion criteria.
- 85% of inadequately controlled studies reported positive findings, compared to 55% of well-controlled studies.
- Dissemination of printed educational materials alone was reported to be ineffective in all adequately controlled studies, whereas every uncontrolled study reported positive effects.

Authors' main conclusions

- Mailed educational materials alone may change knowledge or attitudes, but had little or no detectable effect on actual prescribing behaviour.
- Few well-controlled studies have documented the effectiveness of group education.
- It is not known whether computerised reminder systems could reduce unnecessary or inappropriate drug use.
- Ongoing feedback may be effective in improving certain types of prescribing practices, such as use of generic drugs in academic settings.
- Brief one-to-one educational outreach visits are effective in substantially reducing inappropriate prescribing.

Gurwitz 1990[32] *Impact of interventions to improve drug prescribing and utilisation in the nursing home*

Inclusion criteria:

- Study designs: RCT, CCT, CBA, ITS, BA
- Participants: Not explicitly stated (physicians and nursing staff)
- Intervention: Interventions to change drug prescribing or utilisation in nursing homes
- Outcomes: Changes in drug prescribing and/or utilisation
- Period: Not explicitly stated

Main results

- 16 studies met the inclusion criteria.
- Mixed effects (mainly positive) were observed for all types of interventions.
- Results of single randomised trial of educational outreach were positive.

Authors' main conclusions

- Little evidence available from adequately controlled studies.
- Research needed on clinical outcomes and cost-effectiveness of interventions.

Anderson 1996[33] *Review of techniques to improve prescribing behaviour*

Inclusion criteria:

- Study designs: RCT
- Participants: Not explicitly stated (community physicians)
- Intervention: Interventions to improve prescribing behaviour
- Outcomes: Not explicitly stated
- Period: Not explicitly stated

54

Main results

- 9 studies met the inclusion criteria.
- Printed educational materials alone do not improve practice. Interventions combining education and feedback were found to be more effective.
- Educational strategies involving face-to-face contact between the expert and physician were successful.
- Feedback including specific recommendations for change in the use of medications was more successful than a description of current practice.

Authors' main conclusions

- Specific educational and feedback strategies can improve quality of care.
- Results are limited due to the lack of data found on patient outcomes.
- Need for further research on office based prescribing and on providing information on drugs to patients.

Interventions to improve other behaviours

Grimshaw 1998[34] *Effectiveness of interventions to improve general practitioner outpatient referrals*

Inclusion criteria:

- Study designs: RCT, CBA, ITS
- Participants: Not explicitly stated (primary care physicians)
- Intervention: Interventions to influence the quality or quantity of outpatient referral
- Outcomes: Objectively measured provider performance or patient outcomes
- Period: 1966–1995

Main results

- 4 studies met the inclusion criteria.
- Mixed results were found.
- Training plus structured assessment cards, and joint consultation sessions were effective.
- Development and dissemination of local consensus guidelines and the introduction of fundholding in UK primary care were found to have no effect.

Authors' main conclusions

- Difficult to draw firm conclusions on the basis of this review as a result of the limited number of rigorous studies identified.

55

- Further research is needed on interventions designed to improve the referral process.

Solomon 1998[35] *Effectiveness of interventions to modify physician testing behaviour*

Inclusion criteria:

- Study designs: RCT, CBA, BA
- Participants: Physicians
- Intervention: Any intervention that attempted to modify physician testing behaviour
- Outcomes: Resource utilisation
- Period: 1966–1998
- Other: Only English language studies included

Main results

- 49 studies met the inclusion criteria.
- 76% of interventions reported reduced volume and/or charges for tests targeted.
- 15 of 21 studies aimed at one behavioural factor were successful.
- 24 of 28 studies aimed at more than one behavioural factor were successful.

Authors' main conclusions

- Majority of interventions were successful.
- Trend towards interventions based on multiple behavioural factors being more successful.
- Primary data of low quality hence conclusions are weak.
- Further research should incorporate relevant behavioural change models.

Hanson 1997[36] *Effectiveness of clinical interventions designed to change care at the end of life*

Inclusion criteria:

- Study designs: RCT, CCT, CBA, BA ("Clinical trials")
- Participants: Patients near the end of life and physicians
- Intervention: Interventions to change patient experiences and/or physician practices
- Outcomes: Not explicitly stated (patient preferences, pain control, use of life sustaining treatments and medical costs)
- Period: 1990–1996
- Other: Only studies in USA considered

Main results

- 16 studies met the inclusion criteria.
- 6 of 8 studies (3 out of 5 RCT) of patient targeted interventions (usually written materials and/or discussions with professional or patient representative) to increase the use of advanced directives or proxy measures reported an increase in documentation of patient treatment preferences.
- 5 of 5 non-randomised studies of physician targeted interventions ("sophisticated educational or motivational techniques") to improve recording of advanced directives or use of patient preferences and change in life-sustaining treatments reported positive results.
- 3 of 3 studies targeted at the physician and the patient demonstrated an increased expression of patient preference but showed no effect on the use of life-sustaining treatments or other outcome measures.

Authors' main conclusions

- Several interventions were found to increase the use of patient treatment preferences in end of life care. The success varied with respect to patient characteristics and the educational technique used.
- Educational approaches must be creative and complemented by motivational and organisational strategies to change physician behaviour.

Appendix 4.3 Summary of systematic reviews of the effects of specific implementation strategies on professional practice

Key: RCT = Randomised controlled trial
CCT = Controlled clinical trial
CA = Controlled after
UA = Uncontrolled after
BA = Before/after
CBA = Controlled before/after
XS = Cross sectional
ITS = Interrupted time series

Educational materials

Freemantle 1996[37] *Effectiveness of printed educational materials*

Inclusion criteria:

- Study designs: RCT, CBA, ITS
- Participants: Healthcare professionals
- Intervention: Distribution of published or printed recommendations for clinical care, delivered by hand or through personal or mass mailings

- Outcomes: Objectively measured professional performance or patient health outcome
- Period: Not explicitly stated

Main results

- 11 studies met the inclusion criteria.
- 9 of 9 studies assessing the effect of printed educational materials versus no intervention found no statistically significant improvements in practice.
- 1 of 6 studies observed improvements in care when educational materials combined with another intervention were compared to educational materials alone.

Authors' main conclusions

- Printed educational materials alone were found to have a small impact on practice.
- Additional interventions may increase changes in practice but it is unclear from this review which interventions are most cost-effective in different circumstances.
- Need for further research on the cost-effectiveness of comparing printed educational materials with more active interventions.

Educational outreach visits

Thomson 1997[38] *Effectiveness of outreach visits*

Inclusion criteria:

- Study designs: RCT
- Participants: Healthcare providers
- Intervention: Outreach visits defined as a personal visit by a trained person to a health care provider in his or her own setting
- Outcomes: Objective measurement of health professional practice or patient outcomes
- Period: 1966–1997

Main results

- 18 trials met the inclusion criteria.
- 3 of 3 trials observed significant improvements compared to no intervention.
- 12 of 13 trials comparing outreach plus a complementary intervention with no intervention observed significant improvements.
- 1 of 1 trial found that outreach was more effective than audit and feedback.

- 1 of 1 study observed outreach using patient related content to be more effective than patient related summaries for content.
- 1 of 1 found that effects decrease over time.

Authors' main conclusions

- Effect sizes of outreach visits were small to moderate.
- Support was found for the use of educational outreach visits combined with additional interventions to reduce inappropriate prescribing.
- The cost-effectiveness of outreach visits is unclear.
- Need to monitor long-term performance of the effectiveness of outreach visits.
- More research is required into the effectiveness of outreach visits in different settings and contexts.

Local opinion leaders

Thomson 1997[39] *Effectiveness of using local opinion leaders*

Inclusion criteria:

- Study designs: RCT
- Participants: Healthcare providers
- Intervention: Local opinion leaders defined as the use of providers nominated by their colleagues as "educationally influential"
- Outcomes: Objective measures of provider performance or health care outcomes.
- Period: 1966–1998

Main results

- 6 studies met the inclusion criteria.
- 5 of 6 trials observed improvements in process of care, however these were only statistically significant in 2 trials.
- 1 of 3 trials observed significant improvements in patient outcome.
- 1 trial found local opinion leaders to be significantly more effective than group audit and feedback.

Authors' main conclusions

- Using local opinion leaders results in mixed effects on professional practice.
- It is not always clear what local opinion leaders do and replicable descriptions are needed.
- Further research is required to determine if opinion leaders can be identified and in which circumstances they are likely to influence the practice of their peers.

Audit and feedback

Mugford 1991[40] *Effectiveness of audit and feedback*

Inclusion criteria:

- Study designs: RCT, CCT, CBA, BA
- Participants: Not explicitly stated (clinicians)
- Intervention: Information feedback
- Outcomes: Not explicitly stated
- Period: Not explicitly stated

Main results

- 36 studies met the inclusion criteria.
- Information feedback was most likely to influence clinical practice if it was part of a strategy to target decision makers that had already agreed to review their practice.
- A more direct effect was discernible if the information was presented close to the time of decision making.

Authors' main conclusions

- Information feedback is "necessary but not sufficient in the process of maintaining high quality clinical care".
- The use of information in the audit process should be critically evaluated.

Buntinx 1993[41] *Effectiveness of feedback and reminders on diagnostic and preventive care in ambulatory care*

Inclusion criteria:

- Study designs: RCT, CCT, CBA, BA
- Participants: Physicians in ambulatory care
- Intervention: Feedback and reminders
- Outcomes: Number and costs of diagnostic tests ordered, compliance with guidelines
- Period: 1983–1992

Main results

- 27 studies met the inclusion criteria; 1 study was subsequently excluded.
- 8 studies evaluated the impact of interventions on reducing tests/costs. 2 of 2 RCT assessing reminders and 5 of 6 studies (including 1 of 1 RCT) assessing feedback observed significant reductions.
- 14 studies evaluated impact of interventions on adherence to guidelines: 5 of 7 studies (including 4 of 4 RCT) assessing reminders and 5 of 9 studies (including 3 of 4 RCT) observed significant improvements.

Authors' main conclusions

- Feedback and reminders may reduce the utilisation of diagnostic tests, and they may improve conformity to standards of performance of doctors.
- Reminders appear to exert greater effect than classical methods of feedback.

Balas 1996[42] *Effectiveness of physician profiling (peer comparison feedback)*

Inclusion criteria:

- Study designs: RCT
- Participants: Not explicitly stated (clinicians)
- Intervention: Peer comparison feedback interventions
- Outcomes: Frequency of targeted clinical activity or procedure
- Period: Not explicitly stated

Main results

- 12 studies met the inclusion criteria.
- 10 of 12 studies observed significant effects on various clinical procedures; $p < 0.05$ using a vote counting method; $z = 1.98$ $p < 0.05$ using a z Transformation method (based on 8 trials); and OR of 1.09 (CI $1.05-1.14$) based on a meta-analysis of 5 trials.
- Subgroup analyses of studies focusing on test ordering and prescribing were non-significant.

Authors' main conclusions

- Peer comparison alone is unlikely to result in substantial quality improvement or cost-control.
- Potential cost saving of profiling is unlikely to exceed the cost of profiling for most clinical procedures.
- Need for further evaluation of more substantive feedback and other methods to improve health care quality and control costs.

Thomson 1998[43,44] *Effectiveness of audit and feedback*

Inclusion criteria:

- Study designs: RCT, CCT
- Participants: Healthcare providers
- Intervention: Audit and feedback defined as any summary of clinical performance of health care over a specified period of time
- Outcomes: Objective measurement of health professional practice or patient outcomes
- Period: 1966–1997

Main results

- 37 studies met the inclusion criteria.
- 8 of 13 trials observed significant improvements compared to no intervention.

- 10 of 15 trials found audit and feedback including educational materials to be significantly more effective than no intervention or educational materials alone.
- 6 of 11 trials found significant but modest effects in favour of audit and feedback as part of a multifaceted intervention as opposed to no intervention.
- 5 trials reported mixed results for the short and longer-term effects of audit and feedback.
- 4 trials found little additional benefit of combining audit and feedback with other interventions.
- 2 of 3 trials found that reminders were more effective than audit and feedback for preventive services.

Authors' main conclusions

- Audit and feedback can be effective in improving performance, in particular for prescribing and test ordering, although the effects are generally small to moderate.
- The review does not support widespread use of audit and feedback; audit and feedback should be targeted where it is likely to effect change and should not be used generally for all problems.
- It is not possible to determine the optimal characteristics of feedback.
- Further research needs to consider the effectiveness of combining audit and feedback with other interventions such as reminders, using rigorous designs and better quality reporting.

Reminders (manual or computerised)

Austin 1994[45] *Effectiveness of reminders on preventive care*
Inclusion criteria:

- Study designs: RCT
- Participants: Physicians
- Intervention: Reminders
- Outcomes: Process and outcome of care
- Period: Not explicitly stated

Main results

- 10 studies met the inclusion criteria.
- According to the authors, only 4 studies in 2 areas (cervical screening and tetanus immunisation) provided sufficient data for meta-analysis.
- Odds ratio was 1·18 (95% CI 1·02–1·34) for cervical screening and 2·82 (95% CI 2·66–2·98) for tetanus immunisation.

Authors' main conclusions

- Reminders may increase provision of preventive care services.

Shea 1996[46] *Effectiveness of computer based reminder systems on preventive care*

Inclusion criteria:

- Study designs: Ambiguous RCT and "studies with concurrent controls that also reported comparisons with historical controls"
- Participants: Not explicitly stated (physicians and patients)
- Intervention: Computer-based reminder systems
- Outcomes: Provision of six preventive practices (vaccination, breast cancer screening, colorectal cancer screening, cervical cancer screening, cardiovascular risk reduction, other preventive services)
- Period: 1966–1995

Main results

- 16 studies met the inclusion criteria.
- Computer reminders increased provision of four preventive practices separately and all practices combined (OR 1·77 95% CI 1·38–2·27).
- Manual reminders increased provision of four preventive practices separately and all practices combined (OR 1·57 95% CI 1·20–2·06).
- Computer plus manual reminders increased provision of preventive practices separately for all preventive practices (OR 2·23 95% CI 1·67–2·98).
- No significant difference was found between computer and manual reminders.

Authors' main conclusions

- Manual and computer reminders separately can increase the use of preventive services.
- A combination of manual and computer reminders is more effective than either individual intervention.
- Need to overcome technical issues before the widespread use of computer generated reminders can be recommended.

Hunt 1998[47] *Effectiveness of computer-based clinical decision support systems (CDSS)*

Inclusion criteria:

- Study designs: RCT, CCT
- Participants: Health professionals in clinical practice or postgraduate training
- Intervention: Computer-based decision support system

- Outcomes: Clinician performance and/or patient outcomes
- Period: 1974–1998

Main results

- 68 studies met the inclusion criteria.
- 9 of 15 studies observed significant improvements in drug dosing.
- 1 of 5 studies observed significant improvements in diagnosis.
- 14 of 19 studies observed significant improvements in preventive care.
- 29 studies evaluated the effects of CDSSs on other aspects of medical care: 19 of 26 observed significant improvements in practitioner performance; and 4 of 7 observed significant improvements in patient outcomes.

Authors' main conclusions

- Progress has been made in the quality and quantity of studies of CDSSs.
- Need for larger trials of CDSSs as they are improving.
- Ambulatory care services and clinics should consider opportunities to acquire preventive care reminder systems.
- Reasonable to consider using a CDSS to effectively titrate potentially toxic intravenously administered medications but need larger confirmatory trials.

Other interventions

Sullivan 1995[48] *Effectiveness of computers on primary care consultations*

Inclusion criteria:

- Study designs: "Prospective studies", no further details given (included RCT, CCT, CBA, BA)
- Participants: Doctors or nurses in primary care settings
- Intervention: Computer system to support either routine practice or a specific research project
- Outcomes: Effects on consultation process, doctors' task performance and patient outcomes
- Period: Not explicitly stated

Main results

- 30 studies met the inclusion criteria.
- Most studies showed a neutral or positive effect when computers were used.
- Immunisation rates improved by 8–18%, other preventive tasks improved by up to 50%.

- Consultation time may lengthen up to 90 seconds.
- A reduction in patient initiated social contact may occur.
- An increase in clinical performance by the physician may also occur.

Authors' main conclusions

- Computers in consultation may improve clinician performance but may increase the length of consultation.
- Need for further research on outcomes of care for patients.
- Need for rigorous research to evaluate the effectiveness of existing consultations using computers for clinicians, support staff and patients.

Balas 1996[49] *Efficacy of computerised information systems*

Inclusion criteria:

- Study designs: RCT
- Participants: Not explicitly stated (patients and providers)
- Intervention: Computerised information interventions
- Outcomes: Process or outcome of care
- Period: Not explicitly stated

Main results

- 98 studies involving 100 comparisons met the inclusion criteria.
- 3 comparisons were subsequently excluded due to poor quality.
- 76 out of 97 comparisons observed improvements in process of care (significance not reported).
- 10 out of 14 comparisons observed improvements in morbidity, physiologic or psychological patient outcomes.
- There were no differences across main site categories (outpatient primary care group, outpatient speciality care group and inpatient care group).
- Provider prompts, computer assisted treatment planners, and interactive patient/education therapy and patient prompts had statistically significant effects ($p < 0.05$) using the vote counting method.

Authors' main conclusions

- Four generic information interventions (provider prompts, computer assisted treatment planners, interactive patient education therapy and patient prompts) can improve quality of care.
- Computer systems should incorporate these effective information strategies.

Beilby 1997[50] *Effectiveness of providing costing information to reduce costs by changing general practitioner behaviour*

Inclusion criteria:

- Study designs: RCT, CCT, ITS
- Participants: General practitioners
- Intervention: Distribution of costing information to general practitioners (either as a stand alone or part of a multifaceted intervention)
- Outcomes: Objective measurement of health provider performance, clinical care or patient specific criteria
- Period: 1980–1996

Main results

- 6 studies met the inclusion criteria.
- 2 of 2 studies observed significant increases in generic prescribing or significant reductions in prescribing costs. Printed newsletters and non-commercial drug information were less effective than educational outreach.
- 3 of 3 studies observed significant reductions in test ordering.
- 1 of 1 study observed non-significant reductions on visits to specialists, medical procedures and ambulatory care charges.

Authors' main conclusions

- The provision of costing information can change GP behaviour in all service areas.
- Sustainability of these changes and linking of cost savings to health outcomes have not been well studied.

Grilli 1998[51] *Effectiveness of mass media on the utilisation of health services by professionals, patients or the public*

Inclusion criteria:

- Study designs: RCT, CCT, CBA, ITS
- Participants: Healthcare providers, patients and the general public
- Intervention: Interventions based on use of mass media targeted at the population level aiming to promote or discourage use of health care
- Outcomes: Objective measures of direct impact on health services utilisation
- Period: Not explicitly stated

Main results

- 17 studies met the inclusion criteria.
- 16 reported that mass media were effective; however statistically significant findings were only observed in 7 studies following re-analysis.

- Standardised effect size based on meta-analysis was -1.54 (95% CI -1.12 to -1.97) for planned mass media campaigns (14 studies) and -1.24 (95% CI -0.84 to -1.57) for unplanned media coverage (3 studies).

Authors' main conclusions

- Mass media campaigns may have a positive influence upon the manner in which health services are utilised although current research has methodological limitations.

Shortell 1998[52] *Effectiveness of the clinical application of continuous quality improvement (CQI)*

Inclusion criteria:

- Study designs: Not explicitly stated (single site BA and multi site RCT included)
- Participants: Not explicitly stated
- Intervention: Continuous quality improvement defined as a philosophy of continually improving the underlying processes associated with providing a good service which meets or exceeds customer expectation
- Outcomes: Not explicitly stated
- Period: 1991–1997

Main results

- 55 studies met the inclusion criteria.
- 43 single site studies: most showed positive results apart from the 2 RCT and 2 other studies that showed no improvements in care.
- 13 multi site studies: most found positive results. The RCT found no impact.
- 3 multi site studies are currently in progress.

Authors' main conclusions

- Single site study design makes it difficult to discern if effects are attributable to CQI. Also possible that effects are overstated due to publication bias.
- Quality and outcomes of care can be improved and certain efficiencies achieved. Need physician involvement, individual practitioner feedback and a supportive organisational culture.
- Characteristics of the target condition, lack of physician buy-in, poor dissemination and vague diffuse feedback to practitioners can affect the effectiveness of CQI.

5 Implementing research findings into practice: beyond the information deficit model

THERESA M MARTEAU, AMANDA J SOWDEN, AND DAVID ARMSTRONG

> ## Key messages
>
> Consideration of:
>
> - Implicit models of changing behaviour – passive dissemination of information versus active.
> - Explicit aproaches to changing behaviour based on psychological models – behavioural change based on learning theory versus social cognition.
> - How to determine which behaviours should be changed.

Implicit models of changing health professionals' behaviour

The belief that new knowledge changes behaviour lies at the heart of professional practice. Medical students are transformed into medical practitioners through the inculcation of knowledge; specialist training requires a further encounter with more advanced knowledge, while professional development is built around acquiring the latest knowledge through "continuing medical education". Indeed, when exploring the characteristics of professional status, Freidson identified possession of an esoteric knowledge base, alongside commitment to an altruistic ideal, as marking out a profession from other forms of occupational organisation.[1]

However, the problem with the view that providing new knowledge produces new behaviour – an information deficit model of behaviour change – is that as an explanation it lacks both empirical and theoretical

68

support. For example, in their overview of systematic reviews of interventions to promote implementation of research findings by practitioners, Grimshaw and colleagues noted that there was good evidence to show that passive dissemination of information, such as mailing educational materials, was ineffective (see Chapter 4), a finding echoed in a publication from the NHS Centre for Reviews and Dissemination.[2]

While information may be necessary for behaviour change, it is rarely sufficient, as is illustrated by the consistent finding that patients are poor at adhering to medical advice.[3]

The problems with an information deficit model have been recognised in the education field by attempts to reconceptualise learning as an active process rather than the passive assimilation of information. In this new educational model, emphasis is placed on the learner as an adult who learns by reflection,[4] by problem-solving and involvement,[5] and by self assessment;[6] this model therefore opposes androgogy or adult learning to traditional pedagogy in which the learner is a passive recipient of information. In support of this a recent systematic review provides some evidence that interactive CME sessions that enhance participant activity and provide the opportunity to practise skills are more likely to effect change in practice than didactic sessions.[7]

Nevertheless, despite their greater sophistication and plausibility, adult learning models still pose explanatory and empirical problems. On the one hand, if (adult) learning is defined in terms of behaviour change then explanation becomes rather circular; on the other hand, if "learning" and behaviour are kept separate then the relationship between the two remains unresolved. The finding that a more "active" learning experience is more likely to change behaviour than a passive one still embodies the idea that the problem is one of information transfer: all that changes is the subtlety with which it is transmitted.[8]

Given the specific problem of how to implement the results of research into practice, a number of models have emerged that try to understand the process of changing health professionals' behaviour.[9,10] These models frequently draw on the idea of "active" learning and combine this with concepts taken from descriptive work on diffusion of innovation and technology transfer in other areas. But such models neglect a long tradition within the behavioural and social sciences of understanding and explaining behaviour.[11] The purpose of this chapter is to describe some of the psychological models of behaviour that have been used and some that could be used, as the basis for designing effective interventions to change practitioners' behaviour. While sometimes used to explain and change behaviour at an organisational level, these models focus predominantly upon the level of the individual. Research using such models shows that health professionals' behaviour is subject to similar influences to that of non-health professionals.[12]

The atheoretical nature of much of the research on methods of implementing results of research into practice can be illustrated by the lack of theoretical grounding in studies in this area. We randomly selected 54 studies evaluating interventions to change health professionals' behaviour from a sample of 284 titles in three areas of clinical practice – prevention, diagnosis, and treatment – from the Cochrane Collaboration on Effective Professional Practice (CCEPP) database, now EPOC (Effective Practice and Organisation of Care Group).[13] Three types of intervention were used, with more than one being used in some studies:

(1) provision of information, in various forms, including research-based guidelines, leaflets, and educational sessions (n = 30)
(2) provision of reminders such as stickers on patients' records to prompt the clinician to perform a particular action (n = 29)
(3) the use of audit and feedback, where information about performance is provided over a period of time (n = 5).

Only two of the papers reviewed made direct reference to the choice of intervention being guided by a theory or formal body of knowledge.[14,15]

Explicit approaches to understanding and changing behaviour: psychological models

If medicine lacks a coherent theoretical model of behaviour change, perhaps the problem with psychology is that it has a surfeit! However, despite the great number of identifiable models, two broad theoretical roots – learning theory and social-cognition models – can be identified which provide different explanations for why people behave in the way that they do and therefore offer different approaches to behaviour change.

Learning theory

Behaviourism, based on learning theory, provides an explanation of how behaviour originates, is maintained, and changed. It differs from models of behaviour such as psychoanalysis in emphasising that behaviour is controlled by its environmental consequences as opposed to being the result of internalised experiences of the distant past. One of the main principles of learning theory that has informed many interventions to change behaviour is that of operant conditioning. Once known as the Law of Effect, it states that behaviour which is followed by positive consequences will tend to be repeated, whereas behaviour followed by unpleasant consequences will occur less frequently. A variety of techniques such as imitation, role play, feedback, positive reinforcement, and

70

punishment can be used to develop, establish, or change a behaviour. The behaviourist paradigm requires an analysis of existing behaviour in order to know how to change it; this is often represented by the ABC acronym, stressing the need to understand the antecedents of a behaviour, the context in which the behaviour occurs, and its consequences. The next step of changing behaviour usually involves three tasks: establishing and maintaining a new behaviour and, where necessary, extinguishing the existing behaviour.[16]

Behavioural approaches have mainly been used in psychiatric contexts so that examples of their use in changing professionals' behaviour are few. Payment sanctions as a form of punishment for inappropriate use of injections and rehearsal of communication skills are two instances where a behavioural approach has been effective at changing health professionals' behaviour.[17,18] The evidence regarding the effectiveness in changing doctors' behaviour of target payments and fees for services is methodologically weak. In a systematic review of the impact of target payments in primary care, Giuffrida and colleagues[19] conclude that the evidence regarding an impact is of insufficient power or quality to obtain a clear answer. In another review of the impact of different ways of paying doctors, the limited evidence suggested that paying doctors by salary, compared with fee for service payment, was associated with lower numbers of procedures per patient, longer consultations and more preventive care.[20] From learning theory it is predicted that, given higher quality studies, methods of paying doctors do influence their behaviour, via operant conditioning.

The main criticism of behavioural approaches has been that they treat human behaviour like a Pavlovian dog – get the cues right and change will result. But people are different in that they give meaning to their situations so that a financial reward for one practitioner can seem like an immoral bribe to another. The importance of these individual meanings has been addressed over the last 25 years with the integration of cognitive factors into behavioural approaches to changing behaviour, mainly in psychiatric contexts.[21] This is reflected in the expanded ABC analysis to be ANBC where N denotes emotions and cognitions, thus recognising that it is the perception of events not events *per se* that drive behaviour.

Nevertheless, the current shift away from a view of behaviour as primarily determined by the environment towards one that involves cognition and individual choice has meant that the behavioural tradition has been relatively neglected by psychologists working in general medical contexts. In part, no doubt, this is due to the particular occupational position of the medical profession through which it has gained the power to control its own work. Members of a profession, especially the archetypal profession of medicine, do not work within or respond to line management, especially one that might instruct them to change their behaviour. The medical profession is also protected from the 'external' financial incentives of the market place in that most clinical practice within the NHS is not directly influenced by personal financial loss or gain.

Clinical autonomy is defended on the grounds that it enables doctors to act in the best interests of their patients. Yet over the last decade this justification has been considerably weakened by high profile cases of malpractice and incompetence as well as the considerable clinical variability between doctors that suggests that not all patients can be getting the best possible treatment. The result is a decline in clinical autonomy as more external constraints and incentives are provided for clinical behaviour. These changes mean that there will be increasing opportunity to devise behavioural approaches and thereby begin to exploit more fully one of the most powerful models of behaviour change.

Social cognition models

These models share a basic premise that it is how people think about a situation, a threat, or a behaviour that determines what they do. They differ in the factors they identify as most important in predicting behaviour. Some of these models have been developed to explain behaviour outside of the health context, such as Social Cognitive Theory (Bandura[26]), and the Theory of Planned Behaviour,[22] while others have been developed specifically to explain health-related behaviour of patients, such as the health belief model.[23,24] Three sets of beliefs that have emerged as important in determining behaviour are:

(1) perceived benefits weighed against perceived barriers to the action[25]
(2) perceptions of the attitudes of important others to the behaviour
(3) self-efficacy, or belief in one's ability to perform a behaviour.[26,27]

Put more simply, before changing their behaviour, an individual is likely to ask: is this worthwhile, what do others think about it, and can I do it? There are several examples of the use of the Theory of Planned Behaviour to predict physician intentions and behaviour.[28,29,30]

A further refinement of these models is the incorporation of an individual's readiness for change as a predictor of the likelihood of behaviour change.[31,32] These stages-of-change models see behaviour change as a process and whether someone changes their behaviour depends on where they are in terms of awareness of a threat and motivation and ability to behave to reduce the threat. While such models seem intuitively appealing, evidence that people proceed in a timely fashion along a continuum from awareness to change is currently lacking.[33,34]

The test of the usefulness of all these models is in their ability to inform the design of effective interventions.[35] While these models have been used in tens of thousands of studies to predict behaviour, including that of health care professionals, there have been very few studies in which researchers have attempted to change behaviour by altering cognitions that are predictive of behaviour.[36] While some of these have successfully altered cognitions and thereby behaviour,[37,38] others have found that changing beliefs that predict behaviour does not lead to behaviour change.[39]

Merging the strengths of both behavioural and social cognition models, as has happened in cognitive behaviour therapy, may prove a more effective way of changing behaviour, including that of health professionals.[21] Such a development requires conceptual as well as empirically based work.

Alongside developing methods of changing health professionals' behaviour, conceptual work is need to address the question of when it is appropriate to attempt to change their behaviour.

Determining appropriate behaviour change

Psychological models for understanding and implementing behaviour change are valuable in helping to answer the 'how' question but they do not address the more fundamental question of whether behaviour should be changed in the first place. Never mind the techniques for changing clinical behaviours, what are the "techniques" for determining which behaviours should be changed?

In part the answer is given by whatever passes for authoritative knowledge. Not so many decades ago this was clinical experience and medical history is replete with the failures of treatments introduced because those with wider experience claimed that they did work. Nowadays it is evidence-based medicine that defines the form of medical knowledge that should be implemented, yet even this has its limitations. To take but one example, a study in general practice that tried to implement the trial-based knowledge that warfarin is of benefit to fibrillating patients found that only half of eligible patients could be given the drug: other patients either could not give consent because they were demented or declined.[40] In other words, local circumstances challenged the view of what others defined as "good" clinical practice.

In effect, there is an asymmetry embedded in the notion of changing clinical behaviour. There are two parties, those who wish to change other people's behaviour and other people. But the latter are not impassively waiting to be changed; clinicians whose behaviour is to be changed have their own ideas about whether and how such change might be effected. This means that behaviour change is not a one-sided business, a case of an enlightened intervention trying to change an old-fashioned clinician, but a process of negotiating whose model will prevail and whose behaviour will be changed. For example, those attempting to promote the uptake of research findings might dismiss the clinician's clinical experience as outmoded;

equally, the clinicians might reject the applicability of the so-called evidence to their own work. Indeed, the clinician, through resistance, may succeed in changing some of the beliefs, and possibly behaviour, of those promoting uptake of research findings (which means that a failed intervention from the point of view of the persons trying to change a clinician's behaviour may be a successful one from the clinician's perspective). In other words, the interpretations that professionals place on their own behaviours, such as the information deficit model, might be "mistaken" but are themselves factors that need addressing if interventions are to succeed.

And, of course, these caveats might apply to writers as well as to investigators! The mere writing of this chapter, and indeed the existence of medical journals, can be seen as subscribing to an information deficit model of human behaviour. Information, of course, has functions other than changing behaviour, such as to increase understanding, to amuse, and to give power. As we have argued, on its own, information transfer is unlikely to change the behaviour of the reader but perhaps, if it is coupled with an understanding of how information functions as an antecedent to behaviour and informing cognitions about how behaviour is changed, it may work more effectively.

Acknowledgement

Theresa M Marteau is funded by The Wellcome Trust.

References

1 Freidson E. *Profession of medicine: a study of the sociology of applied knowledge.* New York: Dodd Mead, 1970.
2 NHS Centre for Reviews and Dissemination. Getting Evidence into Practice. *Effective Health Care* 1999;5:1.
3 Miechenbaum D, Turk DC. *Facilitating treatment adherence: a practitioner's guidebook.* New York and London: Plenum Press, 1987.
4 Schon DA. *The reflective practitioner.* New York: Basic Books, 1983.
5 Knowles R. *The adult learner: a neglected species.* Houston: Gulf, 1977.
6 Coles C. Self-assessment and medical audit: an educational appraisal. *BMJ* 1989;**299**:807–8.
7 Davis D, Thomson O'Brien MA, Freemantle N, Wolf, FM, Mazmanian P, Taylor-Vaisey A. Impact of formal continuing medical education. Do conferences, workshops, rounds and other traditional continuing education activities change physician behavior or health care outcomes? *JAMA* 1999;**282**:867–874.
8 Davies DA, Thomson MA, Oxman AD, Haynes RB. Changing physician performance: a systematic review of the effect of continuing medical education strategies. *JAMA* 1995;**274**:700–5.
9 Haines A, Jones R. Implementing findings of research. *BMJ* 1994;**308**:1488–92.
10 Kitson A, Ahmed LB, Harvey G, Seers K, Thompson DR. From research to practice: one organizational model for promoting research-based practice. *J Advanced Nursing* 1996;**23**:430–40.

11 Dawson S. Never mind solutions: what are the issues? Lessons of industrial technology transfer for quality in health care. *Qual Health Care* 1995;4:197–203.

12 Marteau TM, Johnston M. Health professionals: a source of variance in health outcomes. *Psychology and Health* 1990;5:47–58.

13 Bero L, Freemantle N, Grilli R, Grimshaw JM, Harvey E, Oxman AD. ed. *The Cochrane Collaboration on Effective Professional Practice Module of the Cochrane Database of Systematic Reviews.* 3rd edn. London: BMJ Publishing Group, 1996.

14 Wing Hong S, Ching TY, Fung JPM, Seto WL. The employment of ward opinion leaders for continuing education in the hospitals. *Med Teach* 1990;12:209–17.

15 Brown LF, Keily PA, Spencer AJ. Evaluation of a continuing education intervention: "periodontics in general practice". *Comm Dent Oral Epidemiol* 1994;22:441–7.

16 Kanfer FH, Goldstein AP. ed. *Helping people change: a textbook of methods.* New York: Pergamon Press, 1975.

17 Brook RH, Williams KN. Effect of medical care on the use of injections: a study of the New Mexico experimental medical care review organization. *Ann Intern Med* 1976;515:509–15.

18 Kottke TE, Brekke ML, Solberg LI, Hughes JR. A randomized trial to increase smoking intervention by physicians: doctors helping smokers, round 1. *JAMA* 1989;261:2101–6.

19 Giuffrida A, Gosden T, Forland F, Kristiansen I, Sergison M, Leese B, *et al.* Target payments in primary care: effects on professional practice and health care outcomes (Cochrane Review). In: *The Cochrane Library,* Oxford: Update Software, Issue 3, 2000.

20 Gosden T, Pedersen L, Torgerson D. How should we pay doctors? A systematic review of salary payments and their effect on doctor behaviour. *Q J Med* 1999;92:47–55.

21 Hawton K, Salkovskis PM, Kirk J, Clark DM. ed. *Cognitive behaviour therapy for psychiatric problems: a practical guide.* Oxford: Oxford University Press, 1992.

22 Ajzen I. The theory of planned behaviour. *Organizational Behaviour and Human Decision Processes* 1999;50:179–211.

23 Becker MH. The health belief model and sick role behavior. *Health Educ Monogr* 1974;2:409,419.

24 Conner M, Norman P. *Predicting Health Behaviour.* Buckingham: Open University Press, 1996.

25 Janz NK, Becker MH. The health belief model: a decade later. *Health Educ Q* 1984;11:1–47.

26 Bandura A. *Social foundations of thought and action: a cognitive social theory.* Englewood Cliffs, NJ: Prentice-Hall, 1986.

27 Schwartzer R. Self-efficacy in the adoption and maintenance of health behaviours: theoretical approaches and a new model. In: Schwartzer R. ed. *Self-efficacy: thought control of action.* Washington: Hemisphere Publishing Corporation, 1992.

28 Conner M, Heywood-Everett S. Addressing mental health problems with the theory of planned behaviour. *Psychology, Health and Medicine* 1998;2:87–95.

29 Millstein SG. Utility of the theories of reasoned action and planned behaviour for predicting physician behaviour: a prospective analysis. *Health Psychology* 1996;15:398–402.

30 Walker AE, Grimshaw JM, Armstrong EM. Salient beliefs and intentions to prescribe antibiotics for patients with a sore throat. *British Journal of Health Psychology* 2001; in press.

31 Prochaska JO, DiClemente CC. *The transtheoretical approach: crossing traditional boundaries of therapy.* Homewood, IL: Dow Jones Irwin, 1984.

32 Weinstein ND. The precaution adoption process. *Health Psychol* 1988;7:355–86.

33 Sutton S. The past predicts the future: interpreting behaviour – behaviour relationships in social psychological models of health behaviours. In: Rutter DR, Quine L. eds. *Social Psychology and health: European perspectives.* Aldershot and Vermont: Avebury, 1994.

34 Ashworth P. Breakthrough or bandwagon? Are interventions tailored to Stage of Change more effective than non-staged interventions? *Health Educ J* 1997;56:166–74.

35 Fishbein M. Foreword. In: Terry DJ, Gallois C, McCamish M. *The theory of reasoned action: its application to AIDS-related behaviour.* Oxford: Pergamon Press, 1993.

36 Conner M, Norman P. Health behaviour. In: Johnston M, Johnston D. ed. *Health Psychology, Comprehensive clinical psychology, vol 8.* Oxford: Elsevier Science Ltd, 2001, pp. 1–31.

37 Maibach E, Flora JA, Nass C. Changes in self-efficacy and health behavior in response to a minimal community health campaign. *Health Comm* 1991;**3**:1–15.
38 Wurtele SK, Maddux JE. Relative contributions of protection motivation components in predicting exercise intentions and behaviour. *Health Psychol* 1987;**6**:453–66.
39 Weinstein ND, Sandman PM, Roberts NE. Perceived susceptibility and self-protective behaviour: a field experiment to encourage home radon testing. *Health Psychol* 1991; **10**:25–33.
40 Howitt A, Armstrong D. (1999) Implementing evidence-based medicine in general practice: audit and qualitative study of antithrombotic treatment for atrial fibrillation. *BMJ* 1999;**318**:1324–7.

6 Changing clinical practice in the light of the evidence: two contrasting stories from perinatology

VIVIENNE VAN SOMEREN

> **Key messages**
> - Two interventions for reducing the risk of neonatal mortality due to respiratory distress syndrome of prematurity were analysed.
> - The effect of social, behavioural, personal and environmental factors on the cognitive aspects of learning are brought out and their combined effects on the speed with which an innovation is adopted are shown.

Introduction

Diffidence about incorporating new knowledge into everyday practice is widespread.[1] The nature of obstacles to desirable change has been explored and some strategies for changing clinicians' behaviour have been subjected to controlled trials.[2,3] However, the complex interactions between the nature of the intervention and the mind-set of the clinician have received less attention. Here, an analysis is offered of two interventions that produce comparable reductions in mortality from respiratory distress syndrome in preterm infants, but have very different implementation histories. The two interventions are antenatal administration of corticosteroids to the mother in threatened preterm delivery and administration of exogenous surfactant to the baby. Both reduce the risk of neonatal mortality due to respiratory distress syndrome of prematurity by 40%.[4,5]

Methods

The trial data and the history of the implementation of the interventions were reviewed in the conventional way, with computer-assisted literature

77

searches and particular use being made of the overviews provided by the Cochrane Collaboration. Special attention was also paid to the rhetoric in editorials that accompanied new studies. The author reflected on her personal experience of the introduction of surfactant and discussed her impressions of the early days of corticosteroids with more senior colleagues.

Adoption of antenatal corticosteroids (Box 6.1)

In 1969, Liggins reported on the role of corticosteroids in preterm labour in sheep.[6] An unexpected finding was that steroids accelerated fetal lung maturation in the lambs. Quick to realise the potential benefits in humans, Liggins and Howie set up a controlled trial in which 282 women took part, and which was reported in 1972.[7] Although this showed a halving in perinatal mortality from 20% to 10%, the message was diluted by the presentation. For instance, the first results table shows a statistically non-significant adverse effect in a sub-group of 32 pregnancies complicated by pregnancy-induced hypertension.

A large American collaborative trial confirmed that antenatal steroids produced a great reduction in respiratory distress, but failed to find a reduction in mortality.[8] Many sub-group analyses were done and the

---

Box 6.1   Adoption of antenatal steroids for prevention of neonatal respiratory distress syndrome

1969   Liggins:[6] the physiology

1972   Liggins and Howie:[7] the first clinical trial in humans demonstrates effectiveness

1970s Concern about untoward effects[10]

1981   American collaborative trial report[8] confirms effect, but message lost in sub-group analyses
       No consensus on steroid usage in preterm labour[9]

1990   UK publication of meta-analysis confirms effects on mortality and morbidity[4]

1991   Minority of mothers of babies in Osiris (surfactant) trial receive steroids[16]

1995   Uptake still poor, so National Institutes of Health produce consensus statement[11]

---

abstract below emphasises the ensuing negative results:

"The effect was, however, mainly attributable to discernible differences among singleton female infants (P < 0·001), whereas no treatment effect was observed in male infants (P = 0·96). Non-Caucasians were improved whereas Caucasians showed little benefit. Fetal and neonatal mortality ... were not different."[8]

Editorials of the time were cautious. There was much discussion of the sub-group analyses, emphasising that only certain categories might benefit.[9] Fears of side-effects were aired in emotive language:

"The frightening possibilities of long-term harm must be weighed against short-term benefits. Long latent periods associated with aberrant developmental expression are known in the human."[10]

The disastrous misuse of oxygen in premature babies in the 1940s and 1950s was fresh in paediatricians' minds, along with the unforeseen long-term consequences on female offspring of giving stilboestrol early in pregnancy. In addition, artificial ventilation for respiratory distress syndrome, introduced in the 1960s, had become widely available during the 1970s and produced such a dramatic fall in mortality that the steroid effect was perceived as small in comparison and not worth the risk of side-effects.

Perinatal trials were among the first to be subjected to meta-analysis. By 1990 it was finally clear that there was overwhelming evidence of benefit from the maternal administration of steroids when preterm delivery was anticipated. The odds ratio for respiratory distress syndrome is currently 0·51 (95% CI 0·42−0·61) and for neonatal death is 0·61 (95% CI 0·49−0·78).[4] However, clinicians were slow to act on this information. Surveys in the early 1990s showed that only 12–18% of eligible women were receiving treatment. Realising the magnitude of the problem in the United States, the National Institutes of Health called a consensus conference and in 1995 published unequivocal advice to obstetricians, encouraging antenatal steroids.[11]

Artificial surfactant for preterm infants (Box 6.2)

In 1959, four years after the existence of lung surfactant was first postulated, Avery and Mead demonstrated that the lungs of preterm babies dying from hyaline membrane disease were deficient in the material responsible for low surface tension in adult lungs and considered the role of this deficiency in the pathogenesis of the disease.[12] The concept of respiratory distress syndrome of prematurity as a surfactant deficiency disease was adopted quickly. Thus logic demanded surfactant as treatment,

---

Box 6.2   Adoption of surfactant for prevention and treatment of respiratory distress syndrome

1957   Avery and Mead:[12] the physiology
1980   First uncontrolled clinical trial[13]
1980s   Large clinical trials tend to show effectiveness[5]
1990   Osiris trial engages large numbers of neonatologists[16]
1991   UK product licence[14]
1994   Established treatment

---

but there was a long delay before chemists could produce an effective, stable compound suitable for administration to babies.

In 1980, Fujiwara *et al.* reported the first uncontrolled case series in which 10 infants with severe respiratory distress syndrome were given artificial surfactant.[13] The effects were dramatic: the change in clinical condition was so great that in three hours the babies moved out of a prognostic group in which death was highly likely into one in which survival was predicted. All survived.

The preparations that became available in the 1980s were all experimental and unlicensed and the only way surfactant could be given was as part of a controlled trial. By 1991 there had been more than 30 controlled trials, involving over 6000 babies, and meta-analysis showed that risk of death was reduced by 40% by surfactant.[5] Although potential side-effects such as antigenic sensitisation were discussed, there was less emphasis than there had been for steroids. In 1991, surfactant was licensed in Britain and there was a brief period of unjustified anxiety about whether health authorities would fund it.[14] By 1994, enough surfactant was sold in Britain to treat between 6000 and 8000 babies, enough for the 1% of UK babies likely to benefit.

Discussion

Antenatal steroids were first subjected to a controlled trial in 1972, but by 1995 there were still clinicians who doubted their value or worried about adverse effects. In contrast, artificial surfactant was subject to its first controlled trial in 1984 and uptake was virtually universal within 10 years. Why did one intervention take twice as long as the other to become normal clinical practice? The two interventions have similar impacts on the same disease. The two groups of clinicians involved, obstetricians and paediatricians, have similar scientific training and work closely together. However, there are important differences, both in the treatments themselves and in clinicians' perceptions of them (Table 6.1).

Table 6.1 Steroids and surfactant: clinicians' contrasting experiences and attitudes.

	The paediatrician and surfactant	The obstetrician and steroids
Impact on everyday practice of disease	RDS is the commonest cause of death and disability in the neonatal unit	Preterm labour affects a small minority of pregnant women
Disease mechanism	RDS is a surfactant deficiency disease	Preterm labour is multifactorial and poorly understood
Prescribers' views	Effect seen in minutes. Must stand by ventilator as big changes in settings likely to be needed	Paediatricians report lowering of neonatal mortality in annual report
Conflict between two patients	No	Yes
Perception of side-effects	Dismissed too quickly	Lingering possibility of very longterm effects
Pharmaceutical interest	Yes	No
Widespread involvement in trials	Yes	No
Trial technology	Late 1980s	Early 1970s
Opinion leaders' views	For	Against

Everyday practice of obstetricians and paediatricians

For neonatal paediatricians, prematurity and respiratory distress syndrome are the cornerstones of their practice. In contrast, only 2% of antenatal patients will deliver before 32 weeks and few obstetricians spend most of their working week with women in very preterm labour. Thus the disease is a higher priority for one group, who will naturally seek out new information related to it.

Disease mechanisms

Lung mechanics are familiar to all medical students; the physical properties of surfactant had been well established by 1960 and incorporated into the bedrock of preclinical physiology. Paediatric textbooks taught that respiratory distress of prematurity was a surfactant deficiency disease. In contrast, there is no intuitive connection between a serendipitous observation made in fetal sheep and everyday practice in the labour ward.

Immediate impact on prescriber

A paediatrician who gives a few babies surfactant is in no doubt about its effect. He or she must be prepared to alter the ventilator settings within minutes of administration. The effect is obvious and no meta-analysis is needed to convince the clinician. In contrast, an obstetrician who prescribes dexamethasone to a mother does not personally observe any effect. The effect is apparent in end-of-year perinatal mortality and morbidity meetings. An obstetrician responsible for 500 births per year will experience one less death from prematurity per annum if he or she regularly prescribes steroids. One treatment produces effects appreciated by the clinician's eyes, the other by his intellect.

Side-effects and conflicts between two patients

There is widespread professional and lay concern about the side-effects of steroids. The potential adverse effects of antenatal steroids were widely discussed. For the mother there was metabolic upset, increased blood pressure, and increased susceptibility to infection. For the fetus there was all this, plus possible effects on growth and unpredictable long-term effects. Why should an obstetrician prescribe something that had definite disadvantages for one of two patients and only questionable advantages (in the light of the evidence before 1990) for the other?

In contrast, there may not have been enough concern about the side-effects of surfactants. Perhaps this was because the dominant model was of a deficiency disease. The magnitude of the early trials did mean that short-term problems, such as a 4% incidence of pulmonary haemorrhage, were quickly identified and quantified. However, the possibility of longer-term problems due to sensitisation to foreign protein still exists.

Opinion leaders and group pressure

Neonatal intensive care has a short and dazzling history. Ventilation was widely adopted in the 1970s and doubled the survival of infants under 2000 g at birth.[15] The short timescale means that today's middle-aged neonatologists all sat at the feet of the small band of talented innovators who developed the specialty in the 1960s. The British neonatal community is very closeknit and once a view is held by a small number of opinion leaders it will be widely adopted. For surfactant this was a good thing, but other innovations have been introduced before full evaluation.

Obstetrics is a mature specialty with a long history. Obstetricians are more numerous than neonatologists and have more diffuse interests, usually working in both obstetrics and gynaecology. In the 1970s obstetricians embraced technological advance wholeheartedly. Following this they were subjected to criticism from their patients to a degree unparalleled in any other specialty. They are more likely to be sued than other specialists. A cautious attitude to new treatments is inevitable is such a climate of opinion.

Effective continuing medical education and clinician involvement in trials

Less than one in 1000 at-risk mothers treated during the 1980s were enrolled in steroid trials. In contrast, in 1990–91, about 25% of the relevant British preterm population took part in a huge trial.[16] One of the reasons for this vast difference in the exposure of the obstetric and paediatric communities to the trials was pharmaceutical company involvement. Dexamethasone, a long-established steroid preparation, costs £1·00 per treatment course. Surfactant, developed after years in the laboratory, had to be tested in the field before getting a product licence and now sells for about £300 per dose. The pharmaceutical industry was thus prepared to fund large trials.

The advantages of this were that neonatologists had early access to the material and plenty of opportunities to meet to discuss results and experiences. The magnitude of immediate side-effects was easy to assess. Collaborators' meetings were also a forum where such concepts as trial size, confidence intervals, and primary versus secondary analyses were discussed, thus providing excellent opportunities for many of us to learn about evidence based medicine.

Taking part in a well-organised clinical trial involves participants in precisely those activities which are most effective for changing clinicians' practice.[2,3] Participants are sensitised to information about the intervention from a wide variety of sources. They attend seminars which target the subject and are very interactive. They also receive reminders with every patient contact. At the end, they feel considerable ownership of the trial results.

The nature of the trial evidence

Steroid trials were begun in the 1970s. The emphasis in the reporting is on "P" values and whether the differences between groups are statistically significant. The magnitude of the effect is not emphasised. Although there are two large trials, there are also a number of small ones with conflicting results due to small numbers. Even in the large trials the message is obscured by the sub-group analyses. Thus, it was not until the data were subject to systematic review and meta-analysis that the advantages of steroids became clear. When the evidence is confusing, it is easy for highly intelligent people to find scholarly, theoretical reasons for clinging to entrenched beliefs.

Surfactant trials were carried out in the 1980s. Statistical techniques had become more sophisticated. The importance of adequate sample size, reporting on an intention-to-treat basis, reporting the size of observed effects with confidence intervals, and avoiding *post hoc* sub-group analyses were all appreciated. Thus, surfactant trials are easier to read individually than steroid trials and meta-analyses are easier to conduct.

With hindsight, the clinicians who were cautious about antenatal steroids were wrong. Some of the non-scientific reasons are explored above. However, in the 1980's, there remained real scientific uncertainty. What was the meaning of the subgroup analyses? How bad might steroid side-effects be in women with hypertension? What about infection if the membranes were ruptured? Were the trial results still valid in an era of improving neonatal intensive care and falling death rates? Today, with the technology of evidence-based medicine more clearly appreciated, some of these questions could be resolved more quickly. However, the clinician faced with trial evidence will always have to make judgements about whether the trial circumstances match the individual patient's circumstances closely enough that the trial results are relevant *today* for *this* patient.

Conclusions

Neither the nature of the intervention nor its scientific pedigree can fully explain why one innovation is adopted quickly and another slowly. This analysis has shown the importance of clinicians' previous assumptions and beliefs and the cultural framework in which they work. The conclusion accords both with common sense and with academic exploration of adult learning and behaviour.[17,18]

However, the literature of continuing medical education has emphasised the cognitive aspects of learning at the expense of the social, personal, environmental, and behavioural factors to which we are all subject. Clinicians seeking to practise and teach evidence-based medicine must learn to look for the seemingly irrational in themselves as well as in their colleagues. We should consider our previous experience and preconceptions in order to remove the barriers to new ideas.

References

1   Noble J. Influence of physician perceptions in putting knowledge into practice. *Lancet* 1996;**347**:1571.
2   Wensing M, Grol R. Single and combined strategies for implementing changes in primary care: a literature review. *Int J Qual Health Care* 1994;**6**:115–32.
3   Davis DA, Thomson MA. Oxman AD, Haynes B. Changing physician performance: a systematic review of the effect of continuing medical education strategies. *JAMA* 1995;**274**:700–5.

4 Crowley P. Corticosteroids prior to preterm delivery. In: Enkin MW, Keirse MJNC, Renfrew MJ, Neilson JP ed. *Pregnancy and Childbirth Module.* Cochrane Database of Systematic Reviews: Review No 02955, 5 May 1994.

5 Soll F, McQueen MC. Respiratory distress syndrome. In: Sinclair JC, Bracken MB ed. *Effective care of the newborn infant.* Oxford: Oxford University Press, 1992.

6 Liggins GC. Premature delivery of foetal lambs infused with glucocorticoids. *J Endocr* 1969;**45**:515.

7 Liggins GC, Howie RN. A controlled trial of antepartum glucocorticoid treatment for prevention of the respiratory distress syndrome in premature infants. *Pediatrics* 1972;**50**:515–25.

8 Collaborative group on antenatal steroid therapy. Effect of antenatal dexamethasone administration on the prevention of respiratory distress syndrome. *Am J Obstet. Gynecol* 1981;**141**:276–87.

9 Little B. Editorial comment. *Am J Obs Gyn* 1981;**141**:287.

10 Gluck L. Administration of corticosteroids to induce maturation of fetal lung. *Am J Dis Child* 1976;**130**:976–8.

11 NIH Consensus Conference. Effect of corticosteroids for fetal maturation on perinatal outcomes. *JAMA* 1995;**273**:413–18.

12 Avery ME, Mead J. Surface properties in relation to atelectasis and hyaline membrane disease. *Am J Dis Child* 1959;**97**:517–23.

13 Fujiwara T, Maeta H, Chida S, *et al.* Artificial surfactant therapy in hyaline-membrane disease. *Lancet* 1980;**1**:55–9.

14 Halliday H. Introducing new cost-effective treatments into the NHS. Surfactant treatment for premature babies: who cares enough to pay? *Qual Health Care* 1993;**2**:195–7.

15 Cooke RI, Davis PA. The care of newborn babies – some developments and dilemmas. In: Forfar JO ed. *Child health in a changing society.* Oxford: Oxford University Press, 1988.

16 The Osiris Collaborative Group. Early versus delayed neonatal administration of synthetic surfactant – the judgement of OSIRIS. *Lancet* 1992;**340**:1363–9.

17 Nowlem PM. *A new approach to continuing education for business and the professions.* New York, NY: Macmillan, 1988.

18 Bandura A. *Social foundations of thought and action: a social cognitive theory.* Englewood Cliffs, NJ: Prentice Hall, 1986.

7 Roles for lay people in the implementation of healthcare research

SANDY OLIVER, VIKKI ENTWISTLE,
AND ELLEN HODNETT

Key messages

- Greater use of research may come from wider dissemination and clearer presentation of findings in patient information.
- Increasingly, lay people are involved in setting and monitoring healthcare standards and the development and use of clinical practice guidelines.
- Getting research into practice with lay people requires skills for shared decision making in consultations and skills in multidisciplinary working for policy making.
- Learning from implementation initiatives requires lay people to be involved in their evaluation.

Introduction

As patients or potential patients, lay people as well as professionals have a vested interest in ensuring the availability and appropriate use of health care interventions which rigorous evaluations have shown to be effective. However, uninformed or misinformed patients, consumer groups and wider publics can hinder the implementation of research findings. Recognition of this has fuelled enthusiasm for the provision of research based information about health care effectiveness to lay audiences alongside the encouragement of greater lay involvement in health care decision making. It is hoped that informed consumers will expect and demand effective forms of care.

The provision of good quality information to all those involved in health care decisions is extremely important but often not sufficient to overcome the various professional, financial, practical and social barriers to research implementation. In this chapter, we consider some of the ways in which lay people might help to identify and overcome these barriers, and hence contribute to attempts to base health care policy and practice on sound research findings. After a brief consideration of the policy context and conceptual issues, we use selected examples of British and Canadian initiatives to illustrate ways in which patients, consumer groups and others might be encouraged and enabled to facilitate beneficial changes in healthcare. We also consider how approaches to lay involvement might be evaluated.

Policy context and conceptual issues

The implementation of research findings is explicitly encouraged with the movement towards evidence-based healthcare,[1] and policies promoting clinical effectiveness.[2] It is also encouraged by many of those advocating greater patient involvement in decisions about individual health care and greater lay input into decisions about health care policy and practice.[3] Research evidence can be interpreted and used in a variety of ways: some evidence of effectiveness does not convince those who judge care by a broad range of functional and psychosocial outcomes.[4] Furthermore, opinions vary about the role which personal or social preference should play in healthcare decisions. People who place differing emphases on research evidence and personal preference may hold a variety of possibly conflicting views about the aims of research implementation, the appropriateness of different approaches to it, the roles which patients, consumer advocates and other lay groups can usefully play, and the criteria by which implementation initiatives should be judged. The consistent delivery of a particular form of care to all people with a given condition and circumstance, for example, could be seen as an indicator of a highly successful implementation of an effective form of care, or of limited opportunities for individual patients to exercise their own choices.

What roles might lay people play?

Lay involvement in research implementation activities is encouraged because it is believed to add value to those activities and/or because it is seen as politically appropriate. Lay people with diverse backgrounds and experiences might contribute to aspects of research implementation in a range of ways. Policy makers, managers and practitioners who are trying to encourage research implementation might find it helpful to consider three related questions.

1 Who might bring what insights, skills and other attributes?

Individual patients and their carers have particular insights based on their experiences of illness and of particular health services, and may have a strong

87

personal interest in the implementation of specific research findings. Condition specific consumer organisations which facilitate contact between patients, offer information, advice or services, and campaign on behalf of their constituent group can often present the diverse views of their members. Generic consumer organisations working in the health sector, and umbrella organisations of patient groups can ensure that patient perspectives are kept on the agenda and that consumerist principles are not neglected.

2 To what aspects of the implementation process might they contribute?

Lay perspectives might usefully inform, and lay efforts facilitate:

- the prioritisation of research messages for implementation
- target setting
- the selection and execution of activities to promote implementation
- the evaluation of initiatives.

If, as seems plausible, the perceived relevance of research affects its implementation, then lay involvement in research prioritisation and design may also enhance the research implementation effort.

3 How will their contribution best be encouraged and facilitated?

Even if it is not their primary intention, lay people may influence the implementation of research in a variety of ways both while discussing their own care with health professionals and by contributing to decisions about healthcare policy and practice. A few illustrative examples are provided below.

Individual patients in consultations

Interactions between health professionals and patients take many forms, and there are several models describing the different roles which may be played by each in deciding which forms of health care will be given.[5] Clearly there is potential for both health professionals and patients to influence the extent to which health care reflects research evidence of effectiveness. Interventions to influence health professionals' knowledge, attitudes and behaviour have been discussed in other chapters. We focus here on interventions designed to influence patients' contributions.

Various information-giving interventions have been developed which aim either to persuade people to accept a particular treatment option or to help them make an informed choice between options. Opinions about the

88

appropriateness of the two approaches will vary according to the types of decisions and the nature of the options being considered, and with views about the relative importance of research evidence and individual choice. The health care systems within which decisions are made are also important, as they vary with the scope they can afford for individual preferences.[6]

The persuasive information-giving approach has been used with some success in attempts to fully implement immunisation programmes[7] and to encourage uptake of preventive health care services among adult populations.[8] Care needs to be taken to avoid unnecessary anxiety when using such health information to produce beneficial changes in service use.[9] Persuasion can also be seen in efforts to encourage acceptance of generic rather than brand name prescribing. Reminders for patients, and other attempts to improve adherence to effective medication regimes may also be viewed as attempts to implement research evidence.

Media campaigns can also influence the utilisation of health services, although we do not yet know whether the influence is always in the direction intended by the campaign originators nor whether they are equally effective in increasing or reducing service use; nor whether this impact is selective in guiding the use of interventions in those who can actually benefit, or non selective.[10]

The provision of information which explicitly outlines and offers choices between different forms of care is most commonly seen where health professionals recognise there are trade-offs to be made between the benefits and risks of different options. Such information is relatively rare. Most patient information materials are inadequate.[11] They are often inaccurate and out-of-date. They tend to ignore or gloss over uncertainties, and fail to provide reliable information about treatment effects or actively promote shared decision making. A number of tools have been developed for appraising patient information materials according to a variety of quality criteria. The DISCERN tool[12] can be used by patients themselves and by consumer health information specialists. It has been adopted by NHS Direct for "kite marking" purposes.

Even good quality information may not increase patient choice. A systematic review of informed decision making found five interventions based on theoretical understanding of decision making or health promotion which had also been rigorously evaluated for their impact on informed decision making.[13] Together these studies suggest that information and education are relatively ineffective ways of facilitating informed decision making, compared with the context and social influences. Studies reporting manipulation of information (for example illustrations, framing or graphics), and provision of feedback (for example demonstrating learnt skills, or results of a screening test) were more likely to report an effect.

Interactive media have also been used to permit patients to explore a range of options and to proceed through them at their own pace.

An interactive video system for benign prostatic hypertrophy and hormone replacement therapy has been evaluated. Studies show that it is well received and promotes more active participation in decision making by patients.[14,15] Multimedia approaches are expensive to develop and their cost effectiveness needs to be further explored but are likely to be cost effective if provided over the internet to large numbers of patients.[16]

It has been suggested that, in considering shared decision making the issue of problem solving should be separated from decision making. The former involves identifying the single best solution to the problem and the latter involves selecting the most desired bundle of outcomes. A study using these concepts in patients undergoing angiography showed that patients overwhelmingly wanted the problem solving tasks, which required technical expertise, to be performed by or with the clinician but wanted to be actively involved in the selection of appropriate outcomes.[17] Preference for handing control to clinicians was greater for vignettes which involved life threatening problems than for those which involved mainly morbidity or quality of life. A recent review article has discussed the growing, but still sparse, literature on shared decision making and made the case for more high quality research in this area.[18]

In addition to intervening with the provision of information, attempts have been made to encourage people to ask about the effectiveness of treatments which their health professionals suggest and to enquire about alternatives. Several studies suggest that training and role modelling techniques can help patients to ask more questions and elicit information more effectively during consultations.[19,20,21] The extent to which such interventions increase the likelihood of treatment decisions reflecting available research is less clear.

Lay contributions to decisions about healthcare policy and practice

Lay representatives serving on a range of policy and management committees or project teams may find themselves in a position to influence the implementation of research. Most obviously there has been increasing interest in recent years in lay involvement in the setting and monitoring of health care standards and in the development and use of clinical practice guidelines, although practice in both areas has tended to fall short of stated ideals. Lay involvement in audit is officially endorsed in the UK, but it is not yet widespread and lay contributions have, for various reasons, tended to be limited,[22] with many initiatives comprising little more than user satisfaction surveys.[23] Similarly, lay involvement in guideline development has been patchy and of uncertain impact.[24,25]

Patients and consumer advocates have played significant roles in implementation projects. Several of the ideas, examples and recommendations presented in this paper were identified during a workshop convened by the NHS Research and Development Programme in which consumer representatives explored the potential roles of health service users in research implementation and helped set the agenda in this area.[26] (see Box 7.1)

Getting research findings into practice by developing and implementing guidelines has involved lay people in prioritising areas for attention (ASQUAM) as well as involving them in individual projects. Lay contributions are increasingly seen in the development of information materials. In the UK, for example, women from various backgrounds with dysfunctional uterine bleeding contributed to a multi-faceted strategy to promote effective management of the condition by helping to develop leaflets to encourage women to seek appropriate professional help.[27] Focus groups of patients also influenced the content and presentation of a research-based leaflet to facilitate informed decisions about the treatment of cataract.[28] In Canada, the lay member of the Maternity Care Guideline Implementation Demonstration Project in Ontario played an active role in all aspects of the design and implementation of the project, and was responsible for the development of the strategies and materials needed to educate the public about effective and ineffective forms of care. (Anderson, G, The MCGIDP

Box 7.1 Questions to ask when embarking on research implementation (identified by lay representatives)

Who will define the problems and goals?
Who will initiate, manage and fund projects?
Will all stakeholders be involved from the beginning?
At what stage(s) in the process will service users be involved?
Will specific roles for service users be identified?
Which lay people will be involved? How will they be identified and chosen?
Will they be able to express the views of other lay people?
What skills do lay people already have, and what will they need to develop?
Who will set quality standards for monitoring the implementation?
What resources will be available to support lay involvement?
How stressful will the implementation process be for everyone involved?
Will the implementation strategy achieve desirable and lasting change?
Will everyone involved consider the achievements worthwhile?
Will purchasers' contracts subsequently include criteria chosen by lay people?
Will the experience of involving users be recorded and reflected upon for the benefit of subsequent exercises?
Will professionals appreciate the contributions made by lay people and look forward to working with them or their peers again?

Group. Maternity Care Guideline Implementation Demonstration Project. Ontario, Canada: Medical Research Council of Canada [in progress].) People with a genuine experience of the patient's perspective can be vital in helping identify information needs and to ensure that information is presented in an understandable, acceptable and useful way.

Successful partnerships in implementation activities are likely to require early and continuing involvement of people who can speak from the perspective of health service users and are well informed about technical issues.[25,29] The challenges of multidisciplinary working are increased when teams include people who have not been trained as health professionals, as Grimshaw and colleagues observed in the case of guideline development:

> ... inherent professional hierarchies ... and mutual ignorance of different professionals' skills and modus operandi mean that skilled leadership and adequate time are required to ensure that all panel members are actively involved in guideline development. These issues become more important when patients are involved in guideline development groups: the asymmetry of information, the perceived status of health care professionals and the technical discussions involved in guideline development make it difficult for patients to contribute actively ...[30]

Practical, technical and moral support may be required if the contribution of lay representatives is to be maximised. Training schemes have already been developed for the purpose of overcoming some of the barriers faced by lay people trying to participate in activities led by professionals. The Critical Appraisal Skills Programme (CASP) has offered technical training in the interpretation of research reports to consumer health information providers[31] and members of Maternity Service Liaison committees (multidisciplinary groups for discussing and making recommendations about local services). The VOICES project has provided background information about health services management and training in committee procedures and assertiveness to lay committee members.[33]

Lay influences on policy and practice are not always contained within health service or professionally led contexts. Specific interest groups sometimes feel that they must take the initiative themselves. For example, the (UK) National Childbirth Trust has developed its own policy statement about the generation and use of research evidence.[29] Some groups engage in active campaigning activities, either for or (perhaps misguidedly) against practices which represent the implementation of research, sometimes in open conflict with health professional groups.

Evaluation

The effects of different approaches to lay involvement in implementation activities are to a large extent unknown. Ideally lay involvement in implementation needs to culminate in lay involvement in its evaluation. For instance, Portuguese women have helped to design and implement methods of inviting under-screened women in Toronto, Canada, to have Pap Smears (Rael E. Feasibility study. Research efforts to identify and reach Portuguese-speaking women who are underscreened for cervical cancer. Unpublished PhD dissertation. University of Toronto, 2001) and are now members of the trial steering committee evaluating the intervention.

With so much potential for lay involvement to enhance research implementation, we are likely to see more innovative initiatives in the near future. Participatory principles should be matched by clear descriptions and evaluations of processes, rigorous outcome evaluations and critical discussions of successful and unsuccessful initiatives. Developmental work should be accompanied by good evaluative research which draws on professional and lay perspectives from the outset.

Acknowledgements

We would like to thank all those who participated in the workshop held in November 1994 to inform the Central R&D Committee Advisory Group on the Implementation of Research Findings: Bola Arowinde, Jane Bradburn, Alison Clarke, Hafize Ece, Tina Funnell, Hilary Gilbert, Gill Gyte, Christabel Hilliard, Deborah Khudabux, Tara Lamont, Jo Marsden, Becky Miles, Carole Myer, Belinda Pratton, Ann Smith, Monika Temple, Hazel Thornton, Peter Willis.

Some of the ideas incorporated in this paper have been discussed with Amanda Sowden, Ian Watt and Trevor Sheldon.

Ann Oakley and Barbara Stocking provided helpful comments on a draft of the text.

References

1 Sackett DL, Rosenburg WMC, Gray JAM, Haynes RB, Richardson WS. Evidence-based medicine: what it is and what it isn't. *BMJ* 1995;**312**:71–2.
2 NHS Executive. *Promoting Clinical Effectiveness: A framework for action in and through the NHS*. Leeds: NHS Executive, 1996.
3 Hope T. *Evidence based patient choice*. London: Kings Fund, 1996.
4 Oliver S. Exploring lay perspectives on questions of effectiveness. In: Maynard A, Chalmers I, eds. *Non-random reflections on health services research*. London: BMJ Publishing Group, 1997.
5 Charles C, Gafni A, Whelan T. Shared decision-making in the medical encounter: what does it mean? (Or it takes at least two to tango). *Soc Sci Med* 1997;**44**:681–92.
6 Royce RG. Observations on the NHS internal market: will the dodo get the last laugh? *BMJ*, 1995;**311**:431–33.
7 Hodnett ED. Support from caregivers for socially disadvantaged mothers. In: Enkin MW, Keirse MJNC, Renfrew MJ, Neilson JP, eds. *Pregnancy and Childbirth Module of The Cochrane Database of Systematic Reviews* [updated 06 September 1996]. Available in The Cochrane Library [database on disk and CDROM]. The Cochrane Collaboration;

Issue 3. Oxford: Update Software; 1996. Updated quarterly. Available from: BMJ Publishing Group, London.

8 Dickey LL. Promoting preventative care with patient-held minirecords: a review. *Patient Education and Counselling*, 1993;**20**:37–47.

9 Wardle J, Taylor T, Sutton S, Atkin W. Does publicity about cancer screening raise fear of cancer? Randomised trial of the psychological effect of information about cancer screening. *BMJ* 1999;**319**:1037–38.

10 Grilli R, Freemantle N, Minozzi, S, Domenighetti G, Finer D. Mass media interventions: effects on health services utilisation (Cochrane Review). In: The Cochrane Library 2001, issue 2. Oxford: Update Software.

11 Coulter A, Entwistle V, and Gilbert D. Sharing decisions with patients: is the information good enough? *BMJ* 1999;**318**:318–22.

12 Charnock D, Shepperd S, Needham G, Gam R. DISCERN: an instrument for judging the quality of written consumer health information on treatment choices. *J Epidemiol Community Health* 1999;**53**:105–11.

13 Bekker H, Thornton JG, Airey CM, Connelly JB, Hewison J, Robinson MB *et al*. Informed Decision making: an annotated bibliography and systematic review. *Health Technol Assess* 1999;**3**(1):1–156.

14 Murray E, Davis H, See Tai S, Coulter A, Gray A, Haines A. Randomised controlled trial of an interactive multimedia decision aid on hormone replacement therapy in primary care. *BMJ* 2001;**323**:490.

15 Murray E, Davis H, See Tai S, Coulter A, Gray A, Haines A. Randomised controlled trial of an interactive decision aid in benign prostatic hypertrophy in primary care. *BMJ* 2001;**323**:493.

16 Nease RF, Owens DK. A method for estimating the cost-effectiveness of incorporating patient preferences into practical guidelines. *Medical Decision Making* 1994;**14**:382–392.

17 Deber RB, Kraetschmer N, Irvine J. What role do patients wish to play in treatment decision making? *Arch Intern Med* 1996;**156**:1414–20.

18 Coulter A. Partnerships with patients: the pros and cons of shared clinical decision-making. *J Health Serv Res Policy* 1997;**2**:112–20.

19 Anderson LA, DeVellis BM, DeVellis RF. Effects of modelling on patient communication, satisfaction and knowledge. *Med Care* 1987;**25**:1044–56.

20 Butow PN, Dunn SM, Tattershall MHN, Jones QJ. Patient participation in the cancer consultation: evaluation of a question prompt sheet. *Ann Oncol* 1994;**5**:199–204.

21 Frederikson LG, Bull PE. Evaluation of a patient education leaflet designed to improve communication in medical consultations. *Patient Education and Counselling* 1995;**25**:51–7.

22 Kelson M. *Consumer involvement initiatives in clinical audit and outcomes: a review of developments and issues in the identifications of good practice*. London: College of Health, 1995.

23 Kelson M, Redpath L. Promoting user involvement in clinical audit: surveys of audit committees in primary and secondary care. *J Clin Effect* 1996;**1**:14–18.

24 Bastian H. Raising the standard: practice guidelines and consumer participation. *Int J Qual Health Care* 1996;**8**:485–90.

25 Duff LA, Kelson M, Marriott S, McIntosh A, Brown S, Cape J *et al*. Clinical guidelines; involving patients and users of services. *J Clin Effect* 1996;**1**:104–12.

26 Oliver S. *Involving Health Service Users in the Implementation of Research Findings. A report to the CRDC Advisory Group on Research Implementation*, 1995.

27 Dunning M, McQuay H, Milne R. Getting a grip. *Health Services Journal* 1994; **April**:24–5.

28 Entwistle VA, Watt IS, Davis H, Dickson R, Pickard DA, Rosser J. Developing information materials to present the findings of technology assessment to consumers: The experience of the NHS Centre for Reviews and Dissemination. *Int J Technol Assess Health Care* 1998;**14**(1):47–70.

29 Oliver S. How can health service users contribute to the NHS research and development programme? *BMJ* 1995;**310**:1318–20.

30 Grimshaw, J., Eccles, M. and Russell, I. Developing clinically valid practice guidelines. *J Eval Clin Pract* 1995;**1**(1):37–48.

31 Milne R. Oliver S. Evidence-based Consumer Health Information: developing teaching in critical appraisal skills. *Int J Qual Health Care* **8**(5):439–45.

32 Training and support for maternity user representatives. *New Generation* 1995;**14**:(4)22.

8 Implementing research findings in clinical practice

ANNA DONALD AND RUAIRIDH MILNE

> **Key messages**
> - The need for practitioners to acquire and implement new knowledge is contrasted with the difficulties of doing so under normal working conditions.
> - Dissemination of information without the means to evaluate the content is shown to have little value.
> - Suggested means of assessing information and making it accessible to clinical teams are given.
> - Factors that may affect the use of research findings in clinical practice are considered.
> - Sources of information and its evaluation are given.

People must be able to learn and implement new knowledge if they are to adapt to change. Yet it is still remarkably difficult for doctors and nurses in the National Health Service to sift through the thousands of new research findings appearing in the literature and use the relatively few robust findings relevant to their own practice. Current educational methods, from undergraduate training to continuing medical education courses, still rely predominantly upon non-problem-based teaching methods, such as didactic lectures, which do not teach skills for accessing new knowledge. Moreover, the need to integrate research findings into clinical practice is rarely recognised in the provision of ward computing facilities, regional and national library services, or the investment decisions of Trusts or primary care centres.

What alternatives exist? How may we better proceed in future? In this chapter we examine how one hospital firm attempted to implement research findings into practice. We draw from a case study made up from our experience of training clinicians to use evidence over a period of three years. In particular, the case draws from a three year research project, the Front Line Evidence-based Medicine Project, which observed how clinicians coped with using evidence in 18 clinical teams in different London Hospitals.[1]

Case study: Dr Franks' firm

Dr Franks runs a busy medical firm in a London district general hospital. Until recently, Dr Franks and his team made most medical decisions based on previous experience and a modest sprinkling of "the literature". Altogether, he and his team read three medical journals – the *British Medical Journal, The Lancet,* and *New England Journal of Medicine* – for about three hours each week (half an hour each for Dr Franks, his senior registrar, and registrar, and 45 minutes each for the two senior house officers). The two house officers had little time to read anything.

While respectable, the journals did not provide the clinical team with good quality filters of the thousands of articles published each month. No team member had been trained to evaluate published evidence assessing patient care, so they could not apply a rigorous quality filter themselves, nor be confident of their response when presented with conflicting evidence in the recommendations of peers, drug representatives, and conference proceedings. Dr Franks' senior registrar had heard mention of databases such as The Cochrane Library and Best Evidence, which might have provided effective quality filters for information, but the ward computer was old and could scarcely run the Windows program loaded onto it, let alone a large database on CD Rom.

Furthermore, Dr Franks' hospital library and services left much to be desired. The local library holdings were small and frequently missing, the opening hours short, and the librarian friendly but overworked and not trained in searching efficiently for high quality information. MEDLINE back to 1986 was available on two terminals in the library but, due to vandalism, the machines themselves were locked inside a cabinet making it impossible to download information onto a floppy disk. There were no other databases available of relevance to Dr Franks' team and, even if there were, obtaining the full text article involved an inter-library loan that took at least four days and usually a week or more by the time the librarian had retrieved it from the British Library and sent it via internal mail to the ward. Also, as the library was a good ten minute walk from the ward, neither Dr Franks nor his staff used it regularly, nor knew the librarian well enough to know what she might be able to do to improve article retrieval for the firm.

In short, with a case-load of 40 patients at a time, busy takes, and virtually no support for using research findings other than a slow and rather haphazard kind of osmosis, Dr Franks' team was unlikely to do much to upgrade its decision making capacity.

Yet, all team members knew that they needed to improve their ability to upgrade their knowledge on a regular basis. New pressures to stay on top of the latest findings meant that clinicians would need to be much more aware of new knowledge, to improve the quality of patient care; to develop as professionals; and to help the Hospital Trust plan what it needed in the following year.

During the summer, Dr Franks was approached by the research and development arm of his regional office to join a project in which team members would receive the equipment and training necessary to "find, appraise, and act on evidence":[2]

- a new computer (supplied by the Trust), a CD Rom tower that could permanently store and run CD Roms without risking theft
- three databases applicable to general medicine - the Cochrane Library, MEDLINE (back to 1992), and Best Evidence
- basic training in critical appraisal (or literature evaluation) skills from a local trainer (a public health doctor).

The team decided to take part in the project. Here is what happened.

Dr Franks decided to find out more about using research findings or "evidence" effectively in order for him to present the idea to his firm and to other people whose support he would need, including the computer staff, the Trust Executive, and the librarian. Therefore, Dr Franks asked the librarian to obtain some key self-help materials referenced in *The ScHARR guide to evidence-based practice*[3] and enrolled himself on one of the evidence-based medicine courses being held regularly in London and Oxford. Next, Dr Franks began a strategy to have everyone in the team use evidence effectively on a regular basis.

First, he explained to his team at a firm meeting how regular research appraisal or "evidence-based practice" could be of value to them, and asked who might be interested in attending the training sessions in literature searching and appraisal skills. With those interested (all the doctors, one manager, two senior nurses, and one physiotherapist), Dr Franks wrote a short contract committing all parties to a minimum attendance at training sessions and to fulfilment of ward round-based "educational prescriptions" to search and appraise literature at least once a month.

Second, with the allocated regional trainer for the firm, and bearing in mind the firm's schedule of clinics and takes, Dr Franks scheduled four lunch-time and afternoon training sessions, each two hours long. However, without a locum for each session, he recognised that not all junior staff would be able to attend every training session.

Third, Dr Franks' team negotiated the content of the training with the trainer. Together, they decided to spend the first two-hour session introducing the concept of evidence-based practice to the firm and teaching staff to ask specific, "searchable" questions in the literature, the second on finding the best available information in the shortest possible time, the third on appraising the information they found, and the fourth on acting on (or implementing) their appraised findings to real clinical problems.[4] Given the firm's ongoing interest in stroke management, the trainer decided that in the

---

Box 8.1 Critical appraisal criteria for review articles[6]

- Did the overview address a clearly focused question?
- Were appropriate criteria used to select articles for inclusion?
- Is it unlikely that important, relevant studies were missed?
- Was the validity of the included studies assessed?
- Were assessments of studies reproducible?
- Were the results similar from study to study?
- What are the overall results of the review?
- How precise were the results?
- Can the results be applied to my patients?
- Were all clinically important outcomes considered?

---

third session he would ask the team to critically appraise a systematic review on stroke management from the Cochrane Library,[5] using the critical appraisal criteria outline shown in Box 8.1. In this way the training sessions were of real rather than abstract interest to the firm (i.e. they were "problem-based"), and the trainer could concurrently teach the firm the usefulness of systematic reviews and the Cochrane Library as good starting places for efficient problem solving.

Fourth, the local librarian helped Dr Franks to install the Trust-pledged computer and CD Rom tower, and discussed ways of speeding up the process of obtaining hard copies of articles identified on MEDLINE. For the time being, these included the installation of a plain-paper fax machine on the ward with which to fax requests (indicating the urgency of the article) and receive articles. Both acknowledged, however, that the rate-limiting step was the two to three days it took the loaning library to find, copy, and send back the article, which would require major changes to nationwide library services to alter. Hence, for the time being, the firm would rely mostly on the detailed, structured abstracts from the ACP Journal Club database which usually contained all the information needed for making a clinical decision, as well as the shorter abstracts on MEDLINE and the occasional full-text systematic review from the Cochrane Library. The ACP Journal Club abstracts and Cochrane Library reviews were particularly useful as their authors had already appraised and summarised the original articles, thus much reducing the work of the doctors.

Finally, the team decided to locate the computer and CD Rom tower in the doctors' room where it would be both secure and accessible given doctors' unpredictable but real "downtime" between bleeps and long stretches of work.

Unfortunately, Dr Franks did not discuss the project in depth with the Trust Executive before agreeing to participate, and the promised computer arrived with only a small amount of memory, making the large databases too slow for rapid use by busy medical staff. An extra 16 megabytes of memory had to be ordered (costing £150). While the Cochrane Library looked promising, it came without detailed instructions. Therefore, Dr Franks did not realise for weeks that in addition to over 200 completed systematic reviews, it also contained a bank of 140 000 references of randomised controlled trials relevant to different clinical topics, the NHS Centre for Reviews and Dissemination's entire Database of Abstracts of Reviews of Effectiveness (DARE), as well as articles about using evidence and contact numbers for members of the Cochrane Collaboration (Table 8.1).

Despite these delays, training proceeded as planned. Five months after joining the project, Dr Franks and his team were still using the skills they had learnt during the afternoon training sessions. They had found the training good but short, and therefore much enhanced by Dr Franks' newly acquired skills that enabled him to reinforce and clarify concepts on a daily basis. Dr Franks' training role proved crucial given the rapid turnover of junior staff and hence the ongoing need for ward-based training. In fact, the firm was getting a reputation among junior staff as a good place to train, as the critical appraisal skills enabled them to evaluate the literature quickly and accurately, helping them to pass membership exams.

The team also decided to restructure the firm's fortnightly journal club. Rather than present papers based on a loose discussion of their contents, staff began to:

- ask questions they were interested in answering, specifying patients, outcomes, and interventions of interest
- find papers using structured search strategies
- evaluate what they found according to critical appraisal criteria available for virtually all types of medical literature they were likely to encounter. (See Chapter 9)

Table 8.1 Information available in the 2000 (Issue 4) edition of The Cochrane Library,[1] compared with what was available in 1998 (Issue 1).

Information type	Number of entries 1998	Number of entries 2001
The Cochrane Database of Systematic Reviews (completed and in-progress reviews)	358	1750
Database of Abstracts of Reviews of Effectiveness	1626	2698
Cochrane Controlled Trials Register	112 308	290 258
Cochrane Review Methodology Database	398	1349
Information about the Cochrane Collaboration	84	94

[1] The Cochrane Collaboration, Oxford: Update Software, 2000, Issue 4 (updated quarterly)

Obtaining full texts of articles was still a real problem. However, the biggest threat to the project was that the Region could not continue to fund subscriptions to the databases indefinitely. Nor, without a long-term information strategy, could the Trust commit to funding them, although the total cost was small relative to the cost of defending one court suit or buying drugs for a few chronically ill patients. Dr Franks soon began to wish that he had implemented an evaluation process earlier, so as to have some "hard" results to show the Trust Executive. With his enhanced reputation as a clinical trainer, however, and the noise that his staff were making around the hospital about the project, Dr Franks was hopeful that the hospital Trust would continue to fund the databases and maintain the ward computer.

Discussion

Dr Franks' experience suggests that simple diffusion of information, whereby primary or secondary sources of research are given to clinicians without analytical and operational frameworks in which to apply them, is inadequate to ensure its effective use in patient care. Rather, our and others' experience with teams strongly underscores Lomas' thesis that effective implementation of research knowledge requires restructuring of the local environment and coordination of people and resources both within and outside of the firm.

In his coordinated implementation model (Figure 8.1), Lomas identifies three main elements necessary for the successful implementation of knowledge into practice:

(1) the research findings packaged in a digestible form, such as the *Clinical Evidence*, the Cochrane Library, Best Evidence, and the European-based *Journal of Evidence-based Medicine* that provide quality filters for hundreds of primary journals

(2) a credible dissemination body containing influential and/or authoritative members prepared to "retail" the new knowledge, which in this case included the initial trainer, lead consultant, and senior doctors, nurses, and clinical manager

(3) a supportive practice environment, including in this case librarian, and Trust support for ongoing training, database and computer purchase, and maintenance. Without any one of these elements, each of which requires strategic coordination of people and resources, it is most unlikely that Dr Franks' team would be able systematically to implement research findings appropriately.

To these three elements we would add a fourth, borrowed from anthropological literature.[7] This is the concept of "local knowledge" – the local practices, values, and beliefs into which new knowledge must usually be integrated into projects – or risk having them rejected. Our experience

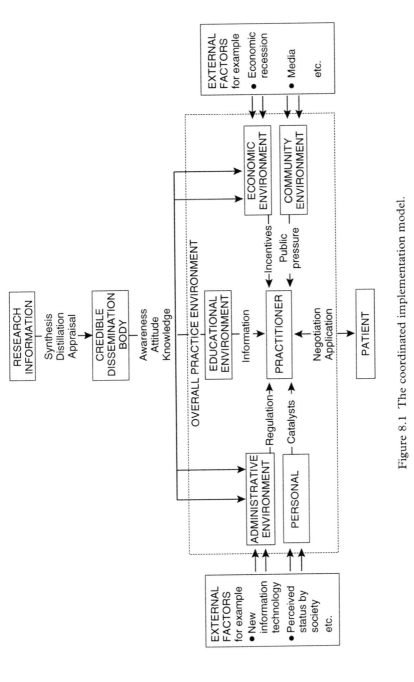

Figure 8.1 The coordinated implementation model.

suggests that systematic use of research findings in clinical practice requires detailed understanding of the needs and environment of the practitioners in question, and that therefore, to some extent at least, each firm's strategy must be developed by firm members themselves. For example, the location of the computer, the structure and content of training, and the allocation of ward round, meeting, or audit time to use critical appraisal skills, need all to be decided upon by team members who alone know what they need at any particular time.

Undoubtedly, however, some needs are common to most hospital firms. Chapter 10 describes how inadequate attention to common potential barriers, such as inadequate skill mix of local users, time consuming bureaucratic exigencies, inadequate information systems, and policy disincentives to implementing research findings in practice, can all result in the failure of otherwise laudable changes in practice. In our experience, addressing these factors, which usually occur at different levels of the health care delivery process (Figure 8.2; Box 8.2), was critical to the success of the firms' projects. Encouragement from management and senior medical staff of the project, time being freed up for clinicians to attend training and implement new problem-solving methods, the use and development of high quality and locally relevant guidelines, readily available sources of information well supported by library and IT staff, and few bureaucratic requirements for organising training and installing databases were common to firms that completed and continued to research findings. Conversely, those firms that delayed or abandoned the project did so for organisational, management-related reasons. These included seniors being too busy to organise and attend training sessions or unenthusiastic about the notion of evidence-based practice and therefore providing no role model for juniors; information sources being too difficult to access (for example, no databases being available within a five-minute walk from the worksite); bureaucratic rules about which type of staff would be allowed to access databases (in some hospitals, only academic staff are licensed to use databases; service NHS staff are not included in the software site licence); no mechanisms to allow juniors

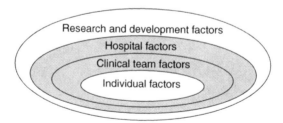

Figure 8.2 Factors affecting the use of research findings in practice usually occur at different levels.

Box 8.2 Factors that affect the use of research findings in clinical practice

	Individual and team factors	Hospital and research and development factors
Enhancing factors	• Dedicated, confident leadership • Ward-based, high speed computing equipment • Good quality databases relevant to the specialty Time and staff support for adaptation period (for example, locums to cover regular staff during training) • Some flexibility in the project to allow team ownership and incremental change • Good relationships between medical and nursing staff • Good quality training relevant to team needs for information • Reasonable keyboard and computing skills	• Services to provide research findings when and where needed: databases, librarian and computing support, document delivery system • Information strategy at hospital level or above • Sustained support for lead clinicians (for example, money for training, equipment, and the development of supra-team projects such as guidelines development; encouragement; coordination with other teams and services) • Good quality training; location; relevance to team needs; sustainability • Good salesmanship and on-site assistance from initiator of project (if external to the clinical team)
Barriers	• Uncommitted leader; overworked; uncertain about benefits; threatened by new approach	• Inadequate availability of research findings: patchy, expensive, non-user-friendly databases; slow or non existent document delivery system; poor computing and librarian support

continued

103

Box 8.2 *(continued)*

- Insufficient external support for training and managing change (money, time, on-site assistance)
- Inadequate computing equipment and databases
- Poor relationships between medical and nursing staff
- Poor keyboard and computing skills

- Lack of management commitment to lead clinician(s)
- Lack of time and resources allocated for ongoing training and adaptation of services around the use of research findings
- Poor training programmes: irrelevant to team interests; one-off approach; impractical to attend

to obtain bleep-free training sessions; and lack of Trust strategies to support those seniors who were enthusiastic but too overburdened with service work to concentrate on developing decision making capacity in their firms.

Our experience suggests that training should not disrupt existing schedules and hence is best held on-site. On-site training also reinforces the message that quality assurance activities should be an integral part of practice, not a one-off activity performed externally by "experts". Training was most effective when it addressed staff's current needs for information and trainers could discuss suitable teaching materials from the outset in collaboration with team leaders. In addition, interactive teaching methods have widely been found to be most effective, enabling learners to refine skills and knowledge that they already possess rather than lecture-based teaching that presents evidence-based practice as an elaborate and alien concept, discouraging newcomers to medical research and epidemiology. Computer equipment must be both secure and readily accessible for busy staff and databases must run quickly, requiring a computer with adequate specifications and maintenance. Existing activities should be harnessed for practising searching and appraising skills, such as journal club meetings, firm and hospital meetings, and ward-rounds, rather than forcing already stretched practitioners to make extra time. Finally, Trust support is ultimately needed for the maintenance of evidence-based practice through the development of library services, the ongoing allocation of time for training, and investment in computing equipment. Such support is an important morale boost to busy clinicians attempting to make major changes to their decision making environments. In this case study, Dr Franks could probably have done more to include Trust board members in the project, for instance by inviting them to an "evidence-based ward round" and discussing the potential of evidence-based practice to the Trust.

However, despite the predictability of many firm needs, Dr Franks' example would suggest that imbuing key decisions with the firm's own local knowledge is critical to gain the credibility, consent, and commitment required to make such changes successful. As Lomas points out, the joint decision making entailed requires considerable coordination,[8] but in our experience, the pay-off is worth it. When allowed to do so, firms have successfully undertaken evidence-based practice in a number of diverse and unforeseen ways, from individual patient care decisions to the development of guidelines and the improvement of local purchasing decisions, accurately reflecting and addressing their different needs and resources.

Acknowledgements

The authors would like to acknowledge all the consultants and their staff whom we have trained, including the clinical teams who participated in the *Front Line Evidence-based Medicine Project*, for making the case study in this article possible.

Postscript (Spring 2001)

Since completion of the *Front Line Evidence-based Medicine Project* in 1998, there have been many new developments in evidence-based health care. These include:

- policies that require clinicians to keep up to date, such as clinical governance and revalidation requirements
- more widespread incorporation of research methods into clinical courses and professional examinations
- new evidence-based health care resources, such as:
  - *Clinical Evidence* (compendium of updated reviews on important clinical topics)[9]
  - National Electronic Library for Health[10]
  - A great many useful websites containing information and tools for using evidence (most can be found by searching for "evidence-based")
  - Many new systematic reviews, conducted by members of the Cochrane Collaboration, as well as by other groups, such as the NHS R&D Health Technology Assessment programme[11]
  - Quality filters on PubMed, the on-line, free version of Medline (http://www.nlm.nih.gov/databases/freemedl.html)
  - *Best Evidence*, which has replaced the American College of Physicians Journal Club database.

Given increasing demand for information to assist decisions by professionals and patients alike about treatments, tests and risk factors, we expect this list to continue to grow rapidly.

References

1 Donald A. *Front Line Evidence-based Medicine: Final Report.* London: North Thames Regional Office, 1998.
2 Milne R, Donald A, Chambers L. Piloting short workshops on the critical appraisal of reviews. *Health Trends.* 1995;27:120–3.
3 Booth A. *The ScHARR guide to evidence-based practice.* Sheffield: School of Health and Related Research Information Services, 1996 (updated regularly).
4 Critical Appraisal Skills Programme. *Orientation guide* 1996. Oxford: Institute of Health Sciences, 1996.
5 Gubitz G, Counsell C, Sandercock P, Signorini D. Anticoagulants for acute ischaemic stroke (Cochrane Review). In: *The Cochrane Library*, Oxford: Update Software. Issue 4, 2000 (Latest version).
6 Gray JAM. *Evidence-based healthcare.* London: Churchill Livingstone, 1996.
7 Geertz C. *Local Knowledge: Further Essays in Interpretive Anthropology.* New York: Basic Books, 1983.
8 Lomas J. Retailing research: increasing the role of evidence in clinical services for childbirth. *Milbank Quarterly* 1993;71(3):439–76.
9 www.evidence.com
10 www.nelh.gov.uk
11 www.hta.nhsweb.nhs.uk

9 Using evidence in clinical practice

SHARON E STRAUS

> **Key messages**
> - Formulate clear clinical questions.
> - Search for the best evidence to answer the questions.
> - Critically appraise the evidence obtained.
> - Apply the evidence.
> - Evaluate performance at all stages of the process.

Introduction

Clinicians need easy access to high-quality evidence for clinical decision making. Questions frequently arise during patient care and occur approximately five times for every inpatient and twice for every three outpatients.[1,2] Traditional sources for this information are inadequate because they are out of date (textbooks[3]), frequently wrong (experts[4]), ineffective (didactic continuing medical education[5]) or too overwhelming in their volume and too variable in their validity for practical clinical use (medical journals[6]). Clinicians are also limited by our inability to afford more than a few seconds per patient for finding and assimilating evidence.[7]

One approach to meeting these challenges is to practise evidence-based medicine (EBM). EBM is the integration of the best available evidence with our clinical expertise and our patients' values.[7] The practice of EBM is a multi-step process as outlined in Box 9.1.[7] In this chapter, we'll focus on how EBM can be practised by the busy clinician.

Asking answerable clinical questions

Every time we see a patient, questions arise about some element of their diagnosis, prognosis or management. In many cases, we will need to track down an answer to our questions and one way to help make us more efficient in this task is to formulate answerable clinical questions.

107

Box 9.1 The five steps of evidence-based medicine

1 Convert information needs into clinically relevant, answerable questions.
2 Track down the best evidence with which to answer these questions (whether from the clinical examination, the diagnostic laboratory, published resources or other sources).
3 Critically appraise the evidence for its validity (closeness to the truth) and usefulness (clinical applicability).
4 Integrate this appraisal with our clinical expertise and apply the results in our clinical practice.
5 Evaluate our performance.

Formulating clear, focused clinical questions requires specifying their four elements:

(1) The patient or problem being addressed
(2) The intervention
(3) A comparison intervention, when relevant
(4) Clinical outcomes.[7]

To illustrate how many questions can arise from a patient, consider a 48-year-old woman who was discharged from hospital two days ago following a cholecystectomy and who arrives in your clinic with the complaint of left calf pain. Dozens of questions can arise as we try to help this patient, and some of them are summarised in Box 9.2 This is not an exhaustive list and indeed, there are many other types of questions that could be asked when considering this patient. Given their breadth and number, and admitting that we are likely to have only about 30 minutes in the next week to address any of them,[8] we need to pare all of these down to just one question. Factors to consider when deciding which question to answer first include:

• Which question is most important to the patient's well being?
• Which question is most relevant to our learners' needs?
• Which question is most feasible to answer within the time we have available?
• Which question is most interesting?
• Which question is most likely to recur in our practice?[7]

For our patient we decide to focus on the question, in a patient with suspected deep vein thrombosis are there any features on history or clinical examination that can be used to rule in or rule out the diagnosis of deep vein thrombosis?

Box 9.2   Examples of clinical questions that arise from our patient

Clinical findings: In a patient with suspected DVT, what is the most accurate and precise way of diagnosing DVT on clinical examination?

Aetiology: In a patient with DVT, can use of oral contraceptives cause DVT?

Differential diagnosis: In a patient with calf pain, what is the most likely cause, deep vein thrombosis or a ruptured Baker's cyst?

Diagnostic tests: In a patient with suspected DVT, can the use of the clinical examination and compression ultrasound rule out the diagnosis of DVT?

Prognosis: In a patient with DVT, what is the risk of developing post-thrombotic syndrome?

Therapy: In a patient with DVT, can she be anticoagulated with low molecular weight heparin safely on an outpatient basis as compared to receiving therapy on an inpatient service?

Prevention: In patients undergoing major abdominal surgery, does prophylaxis with subcutaneous heparin during the perioperative period decrease the risk of DVT?

Searching for the best evidence

After we have developed our question, we need to identify the best evidence with which we can answer it. Finding an answer to our question includes selecting an appropriate evidence resource and executing a search strategy. The types and numbers of evidence resources are rapidly expanding and some of them have already undergone critical appraisal. Many of the available evidence resources are outlined in Chapter 3 (Box 3.1) but a few will be highlighted in this chapter. For example, a new generation of textbooks is being developed whereby rigorous methodological criteria are used to systematically retrieve, appraise and summarise evidence. *Clinical Evidence* published by BMJ Books provides high-quality evidence in a user-friendly format and is available both as a paper version and online. The other useful feature of this resource is that the material is updated twice yearly. This is a tremendous improvement over traditional textbooks in which the material is out-of-date by the time that the book is published.[3]

The most rigorous of the preappraised sources are the systematic reviews of the effects of health care generated by the Cochrane Collaboration and available as the *Cochrane Library*.[9] These reviews are contained in one of 4 databases provided by the *Cochrane Library* that also includes the Cochrane Controlled Trials Registry, the largest database of controlled trials.

Clinical articles about diagnosis, prognosis, therapy, etiology, quality of care and economics that pass both specific methodological standards (such that their results are likely to be valid) and clinical scrutiny for relevance appear in evidence-based journals of secondary publication such as *ACP Journal Club, Evidence Based Medicine* and the *Journal of Evidence-based Health Care*. The contents of *ACP Journal Club* and *Evidence-Based Medicine* are also available online and on a CD (Best Evidence).

If the foregoing rapid, evidence access strategies do not yield an answer to our question, we can turn to the time-honoured and increasingly friendly systems for searching the primary medical literature via MEDLINE and EMBASE employing methodological quality filters to maximise the yield of high quality evidence. PubMed is one interface that allows us to search MEDLINE and its Clinical Queries function provides access to some of these search filters. Using the terms "deep vein thrombosis" and "clinical model" we found a 1995 article in both the Cochrane Library and Best Evidence which describes a clinical prediction rule for diagnosing deep vein thrombosis.[10] Using the same terms while searching PubMed in the Clinical Queries mode identified a 1999 article describing a validation of this clinical decision rule.[11] We decide that this latter reference looks relevant to our clinical question.

Critically appraising the evidence

Once we find potentially useful evidence, we have to critically appraise it and determine if it is valid, important and applicable to our patients. Guides have been generated to help us evaluate the validity of evidence from various study types including evidence about diagnostic tests,[12] therapy,[13] guidelines[14] and clinical prediction rules[15] and some of these guides are also available online [www.cche.net]. With the gradual acceptance of the "more informative abstract", many of the guides can be answered from reading it.

Assessing the article that we found, we can determine that it meets most of the criteria for valid decision rules and note that a clinical model including nine items on the history and physical examination can be used to accurately classify patients with suspected deep vein thrombosis into low, moderate and high probability groups. Using the model, our patient scores one point for having had recent major surgery and one point for having localised tenderness along the distribution of the deep venous system.[11] According to the decision rule, our patient has a moderate pre-test probability of a DVT and it suggest that we should start her on heparin and arrange for a compression ultrasound. If the ultrasound is positive, we treat her for a DVT and if it is negative, we repeat the ultrasound in 1 week.

After we have gone to the trouble of finding an article and determining if its results are valid and useful, it often would be helpful to file our summary so that we can refer to it again or pass it along to colleagues or other learners.

110

One way to do this is to prepare a one-page summary of the patient, the evidence and the clinical bottom line, organised as a critically appraised topic or CAT.[16] There are many websites available that contain CAT databases but before clinicians use them, they should determine what peer review process they were subjected to. From the Users' Guide for assessing clinical decision rules[15] we also find a website [http://med. mssm.edu/ebm] that provides a calculator for deriving the post-test probability for patients with suspected DVT using the results of the clinical decision rule that we found which will enable us to use the study easily in clinic.

Applying the evidence

Applying the results of our critical appraisal involves integrating our own clinical expertise and our knowledge of the unique features of our patients and their circumstances and expectations. Box 9.3 outlines some of the questions to consider when deciding on the applicability of evidence.[17] In determining applicability, we need to decide if our patient is so different from those included in the study that its results cannot help in the management of our patient. The answer to this question is usually no because differences between our patients and those in the trials tend to be quantitative (matters of degree in risk or responsiveness) rather than qualitative (no response or adverse response to therapy).[17]

Box 9.3. Applicability of the evidence

1 Is my patient so different from those in the study that its results cannot be applied to my patient?
2 What are the likely benefits and harms for my patient?
3 Is this intervention/diagnostic test available in my setting?
4 How will my patient's values influence the decision?

When considering our patient, we need to determine if serial ultrasonography is available in our community and if our patient is willing to agree to this management plan. If this is not available, we may need to consider proceeding directly to venography.

Evaluation of our performance

Evaluation of these four steps to practising EBM completes the cycle. We can evaluate our progress through each stage of asking answerable questions (were they?), searching for the best evidence (did we find good evidence quickly?), critical appraisal (did we do so effectively and efficiently?), and integrating the appraisal with our clinical expertise and our patient's unique values and circumstances (did we end up with a rational, acceptable management strategy?). This fifth step of self-evaluation allows us to focus on earlier steps that need improvement in the future. We can assess our application of the evidence we found about the clinical decision model for DVT and decide whether we could have done a more efficient search.

Can clinicians actually practise EBM?

It is useful to distinguish three different ways in which clinicians incorporate evidence into their practices. First is the "doing" mode in which at least the first four steps of EBM are carried out before an intervention is offered.[18] Second is the "using" mode in which searches are restricted to evidence sources that already have undergone critical appraisal by others, such as abstracts from *ACP Journal Club*. Third is the replicating mode, exhibited by clinicians who either do not yet have decision making power (such as housestaff) or abdicate it in favour of replicating the decision of authorities who might or might not incorporate evidence into their decision making. However, even clinicians trained in the "doing" mode move back and forth between these modes, typically depending on whether they are dealing with clinical problems they encounter frequently or only rarely.

Clinicians recognise working in these various modes. In a survey of UK general practitioners, the majority reported practising at least part of their time in the "using" mode using evidence-based summaries generated by others.[19] In contrast, fewer claimed to understand (and to be able to explain) the appraising tools of number needed to treat (NNTs) and confidence intervals.

Can clinicians get at the evidence quickly enough to use it on a busy clinical service? Some evidence is available to suggest that this is possible.[20] One study found that electronic summaries of pre-appraised evidence could be accessed in 10 to 25 seconds[20] and this evidence had an impact on the management of patients.

Once they get the evidence, can clinicians provide evidence-based care to their patients? Encouraging results have been found in clinical audits carried out in various settings. These audits show that the attainment of evidence-based practice is possible in busy clinical settings.[21-26]

Conclusions

Practising EBM is one way for us to keep up to date with the exponentially growing medical literature, not just by more efficient "browsing" but by improving our skills in asking answerable questions, finding the best evidence, critically appraising it, integrating it with our clinical expertise and our patients' values and applying the results in our clinical practice. When added to conscientiously practised clinical skills and constantly developing clinical expertise, sound external evidence can efficiently and effectively be brought to bear on our patients' problems.

References

1 Osheroff JA, Forsythe DE, Buchanan BG *et al.* Physicians' information needs: analysis of questions posed during clinical teaching. *Ann Intern Med* 1991;**114**:576–81.
2 Covell DG, Uman GC, Manning PR. Information needs in office practice: are they being met? *Ann Intern Med* 1985;**103**:596–9.
3 Antman EM, Lau J, Kupelnick B *et al.* A comparison of results of meta-analyses of randomised control trials and recommendations of clinical experts. *JAMA* 1992;**268**:240–8.
4 Oxman A, Guyatt GH. The science of reviewing research. *Ann NY Acad Sci* 1993;**703**:125–34.
5 Davis D, O'Brien MA, Freemantle N *et al.* Impact of formal continuing medical education: do conferences, workshops, rounds and other traditional continuing education activities change physician behavior or health care outcomes? *JAMA* 1999;**282**:867–74.
6 Haynes RB. Where's the meat in clinical journals [editorial]? *ACP JC* 1993;**119**:A22–23.
7 Sackett DL, Straus SE, Richardson WS, Rosenberg W, Haynes RB. *Evidence-Based Medicine: How to practise and teach it.* London: Churchill Livingstone, 2000.
8 Sackett DL. Using evidence-based medicine to help physicians keep up to date. *Serials* 1996;**9**:178–81.
9 *Cochrane Library.* Oxford: Update Software.
10 Wells PS, Hirsh J, Anderson DA *et al.* Accuracy of clinical assessment of deep vein thrombosis. *Lancet* 1995;**345**:1326–30.
11 Anderson DA, Wells PS, Stiell I *et al.* Thrombosis in the emergency department. *Arch Intern Med* 1999;**159**:477–82.
12 Jaeschke R, Guyatt GH, Sackett DL for the Evidence-Based Medicine Working Group. Users' Guides to the Medical Literature: How to read an article about diagnosis. *JAMA* 1994;**271**:389–91.
13 Guyatt GH, Sackett DL, Cook DJ for the Evidence-Based Medicine Working Group. Users' Guides to the Medical Literature: How to use an article about therapy or prevention. *JAMA* 1994;**271**:59–63.
14 Hayward RS, Wilson M, Tunis S *et al.* for the Evidence-Based Medicine Working Group. Users' Guides to the Medical Literature: How to use an article about clinical practice guidelines. *JAMA* 1995;**274**:570–4.
15 McGinn TG, Guyatt GH, Wyer PC *et al.* for the Evidence-Based Medicine Working Group. Users' Guides to the Medical Literature: How to use articles about clinical decision rules. *JAMA* 2000;**284**:79–84.
16 Sauve J-S, Lee HN, Meade MO *et al.* and the General Internal Medicine Fellowship Programme of McMaster University. The critically-appraised topic (CAT): a resident-initiated tactic for applying users' guides at the bedside. *Ann R Coll Phys Surg* 1995;**28**:396–8.
17 Glasziou P, Guyatt GH, Dans A *et al.* Applying the results of trials and systematic reviews to individual patients. *ACP JC* 1998;**129**:A15–16.
18 Straus SE, McAlister FA. Evidence-Based Medicine: A commentary on common criticisms. *CMAJ* 2000;**163**:837–9.
19 McColl A, Smith H, White P, Field J. General practitioners' perceptions of the route to evidence based medicine: a questionnaire survey. *BMJ* 1998;**316**:361–5.
20 Sackett DL, Straus SE. Finding and applying evidence during clinical rounds: the 'evidence cart'. *JAMA* 1998;**280**:1336–8.

21 Ellis J, Mulligan I, Rowe J, Sackett DL. Inpatient general medicine is evidence based. *Lancet* 1995;**346**:407–10.
22 Geddes JR, Game D, Jenkins NE, Peterson LA, Pottinger GR, Sackett DL. What proportion of primary psychiatric interventions are based on randomised evidence? *Qual Health Care* 1996;**5**:215–17.
23 Gill P, Dowell AC, Neal RP, Smith N, Heywood P, Wilson AK. Evidence-based general practice: a retrospective study of interventions in our training practice. *BMJ* 1996;**312**:819–21.
24 Kenny SE, Shankar KR, Rentala R, Lamont GL, Lloyd DA. Evidence-based surgery: interventions in a regional paediatric surgical unit. *Arch Dis Child* 1997;**76**:50–3.
25 Baraldini V, Spitz L, Pierro A. Evidence-based operations in paediatric surgery. *Pediatr Surg Int* 1998;**13**:331–5.
26 Howes N, Chagla L, Thorpe M, McCullough P. Surgical practice is evidence-based. *Br J Surg* 1997;**84**:1220–3.

10 Barriers and bridges to evidence-based clinical practice

BRIAN HAYNES AND ANDREW HAINES

Key messages

- Barriers to changing practice may occur at a number of points along the pathway from evidence generation to clinical application.
- Barriers can be overcome using a variety of approaches depending on where in the pathway they occur.

Introduction

Clinicians and healthcare planners seeking to improve the quality and efficiency of health services can find help from evidence from healthcare research. This evidence is increasingly accessible through information services combining high quality evidence with information technology. But there are several important barriers to the successful application of evidence from research. This chapter will outline both the prospects for harnessing evidence to improve health care and the problems that readers – clinicians, planners, and patients – will need to overcome to enjoy the benefits (Box 10.1).

The aim of evidence-based health care is to provide the means by which current best evidence from research can be judiciously and conscientiously applied in the prevention, detection, and care of human health disorders.[1] This aim is decidedly ambitious, given how slowly important new treatments disseminate into practice[2-4] and how resistant existing treatments that have been debunked or superseded are to being removed from practice.[5]

The barriers to dissemination and timely application of evidence in healthcare decision making are complex and poorly understood. They include many factors beyond the control of the practitioner and patient (such as being in the wrong place when illness comes) as well as factors that might be modified to advantage (such as doing the wrong thing at the

Box 10.1   Some barriers to evidence-based clinical practice and some solutions

Barriers

- the size and noise of the research enterprise
- problems in developing evidence-based clinical policy
- difficulties in applying evidence in practice, including
  - poor access to current best evidence and guidelines
  - organisational barriers
  - ineffectual continuing education
  - low patient adherence to treatments
  - lack of access to cost effective medications or other interventions

Solutions

- research abstraction and synthesis services
- guidelines for guidelines
- information systems that integrate evidence and guidelines with patient care
- facilities and incentives for effective care; disease management systems
- effective continuing education and quality improvement programs for practitioners
- effective strategies to assist patients to follow evidence-based health care advice
- increased resources and essential drug policies

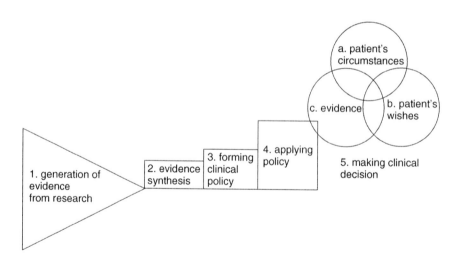

Figure 10.1 Path from evidence generation to clinical application.

right time). Rather than attempt to dissect all these barriers, we present a simple path (Figure 10.1) along which evidence might travel to assist with healthcare decisions in a timely way. We will consider both some barriers along this path and some bridges that are being constructed over the barriers.

116

The research wedge (step 1)

The path begins (see Figure 10.1, step 1) with a wedge that represents biomedical research, the process of testing innovations in health care, eliminating those that lack merit (thus, the shape of the wedge). Testing of innovations begins at the broad edge of the wedge, usually in laboratories, with many new products and processes failing and being discarded on early testing. Those with merit in early testing then undergo field trials in humans, these studies being first aimed at assessing tolerability and major toxicity, then at estimating efficacy. Again, many innovations fail, but a few merit more definitive testing in large controlled trials with major clinical end-points. It is only when studies show success at the tip of the wedge that major efforts at dissemination and application are warranted. Increasingly, behavioural interventions, surgical procedures, and alternative approaches to the organization and delivery of care are being subjected to similarly rigorous evaluation.

The biomedical and applied research enterprise represented by the wedge is vigorous, with an estimated annual investment in 1996 of over US $55 billion around the world,[6] giving rise to the hope that health care can be improved despite cutbacks in health service spending in many countries. Unfortunately, many loose connections exist between the research effort and clinical practice, not the least of which is that preliminary studies far outnumber definitive ones, and all compete in the medical literature and other media for the attention of readers.[7]

Steps from research to practice

The boxes following the wedge in Figure 10.1 (steps 2–4) represent three steps that are needed to harness research evidence for healthcare practice. These steps include 2 – getting the evidence straight, 3 – developing clinical policy from the evidence, and 4 – applying the policy at the right place, way, and time. All three steps must be negotiated to form a valid connection between evidence and practice.

Getting the evidence straight (step 2)

Most news from research appears first in peer-reviewed journals, but the small number of clinically important studies is thinly spread throughout a vast literature, so that individual readers are bound to be overwhelmed. Skills in critical appraisal of evidence have been developed and disseminated for some time[8] but applying these is time-consuming. Bridges for this barrier include abstract services that apply principles of critical appraisal to select studies that are ready for clinical application, and independently summarize

117

these studies.[9,10] Many more of these "new breed" journals are in development so that eventually most major clinical specialties will have their own. More important, the Cochrane Collaboration has pledged to summarise all sound trials of healthcare interventions and the *Cochrane Library* is now a robust resource.[11] Even more recently, *Clinical Evidence*, a twice yearly publication, has set a new standard for summarizing and integrating the best relevant research related to specific healthcare problems (*Clinical Evidence. A compendium of the best available evidence for effective health care*. London: BMJ Publishing Group. Serial publication: www.clinicalevidence.org.).

Along with these new services, advances in information technology now provide quick and often very inexpensive access to high quality healthcare evidence from the bedside, office, and home.[8,12] The most advanced of these electronic evidence-based services is *Ovid's Evidence-Based Medicine Reviews* (OVID Technologies Inc, New York, NY., www.ovid.com), which includes and links *Best Evidence* (the cumulated contents of *ACP Journal Club* and *Evidence-Based Medicine*), *The Cochrane Library*, and *Clinical Evidence*, with traditional large medical literature databases, such as MEDLINE and EMBASE, and fulltext journal access for over 400 journals. Computerised decision support systems, which link "best practices" evidence with individual patients, are now maturing and taking evidence one step further, working it into patient-specific reminders and decision aids embedded in clinical information systems (see Chapter 11).[13] These innovations are making evidence-based health care much more feasible.

Creating evidence-based clinical policy (step 3)

To be both evidence-based and clinically useful, clinical policy must carefully balance the strengths and limitations of all relevant research evidence with the practical realities of the healthcare and clinical setting.[14] This is a problematic step at present because of limitations in both evidence and policy making. Clinical practice guidelines derived by national groups can help individual practitioners, but the expertise, will, resources, and effort required to make them scientifically sound as well as clinically helpful are in short supply, as witnessed by conflicting guidelines from various august bodies.[15] National healthcare policies are often moulded by a range of non-research factors, including historical, cultural, and ideological influences. Moreover, when national guidelines or healthcare policies exhort clinicians to perform acts that are not evidence-based, this unnecessary work acts as a barrier to implementation of well-founded knowledge. "Guidelines for guidelines" have been developed that will help if followed.[16]

Evidence and guidelines must be understood by practitioners if they are to be well applied, a slow process that is not much aided by traditional continuing education offerings.[17] Further, local and individual clinical practice circumstances often vary for the delivery of care, and national guidelines must be tailored for local circumstances by local practitioners if they are to be applied, a process that is only just beginning to occur.[18] Evidence can be used directly by individual practitioners to make policies, but few practitioners have the time and skill to do so. The difficulties in developing sound policies are perhaps the greatest barriers to implementation of research findings at present. Clinicians are in the best position to be able to balance research evidence with clinical circumstances, and must think and act as part of the planning team if progress is to be made.

Applying evidence-based policy in practice (step 4)

The next step from research to practice is to apply evidence-based policy at the right time and place and in the right way. Again there are barriers at the local and individual clinical levels. For example, for thrombolysis for acute myocardial infarction to be delivered within its brief time window of efficacy, the patient must recognise the symptoms, get to the hospital (avoiding a potentially delaying call to his/her family physician), and be seen right away by a health professional who recognises the problem and initiates treatment. For many people in many places, this is still not happening.[19] Meanwhile, newer evidence shows that immediate percutaneous transluminal angioplasty is generally superior to thrombolysis,[20] emphasising both that "current best treatment" continues to change and that decisions to implement new technology must be made in the light of available resources and with the means to address resource problems that new treatments usually raise.

In some cases, particularly for surgery and other skilled procedures, lack of training constitutes a barrier. The complexity of guidelines may also thwart their application.[21] Organisational barriers to change must also be dealt with, for example ensuring that general practitioners have access to echocardiography for the diagnosis of heart failure before starting angiotensin-converting enzyme inhibitors in patients with suggestive signs and symptoms.[22]

Changes in the organisation of care, including disease management, patient-centred care, improvements in continuing education and quality improvement interventions for practitioners,[17] and advances in computerised decision support systems,[13] are beginning to make inroads into these last steps of connecting research evidence with practice. Unfortunately, these may all be undermined by limitations in resources for health services, and the use of inappropriate economic measures for evaluating healthcare programmes[23] when cost-effective interventions may require considerable upfront investment with delayed benefits, as is especially true for preventive procedures.

Making clinical decisions (step 5)

Once the evidence has been delivered to the practitioner and the practitioner has recalled the evidence correctly and at the right place and time, there are still steps to be taken. First, the practitioner must determine the patient's unique circumstances: how is the problem affecting this patient? For example, the cost-effectiveness of lowering cholesterol with statins is highly dependent on the patient's own risk of adverse outcomes.[24] What other problems is the patient suffering from that might bear on which treatments are likely to be safe and effective? For example, carotid endarterectomy is highly effective for symptomatic, tight carotid stenosis[25] but patients must be surgically fit to receive it. Sizing up the patient's clinical circumstances is the domain of clinical expertise, without which no amount of evidence from research will suffice.

Also, and increasingly, the patient's preferences, values, and rights are entering into the process of deciding on the appropriate management. Thus, patients who are averse to immediate risk or cost may decline surgical procedures that offer longer-term benefits, including endarterectomy, even if they are surgically fit. Evidence from research must be integrated with the patient's clinical circumstances and wishes to derive a meaningful decision about management, a process that no "cookbook" can describe. Indeed, we are still ignorant about the art of clinical practice. Although there is some evidence that exploring patients' experiences of illness may lead to improvements in their outcomes,[26] the topic of improving communication between clinician and patient is in need of major research efforts if we are to enhance progress in achieving evidence-based health care. Meanwhile, there is a growing body of information for patients that is both scientifically sound and intelligible, and many consumer and patient groups have made such material widely available.[27] Interactive media are being employed (but are not widely deployed) to assist patients with diagnostic and treatment choices.[28,29]

Finally, patients must follow the prescribed treatment, increasingly on their own because of success in developing effective treatments that allow ambulatory, self-administered care and in some countries cutbacks in health services that necessitate more self-care. At present, we can help patients stay in care, but we are not so successful in helping them follow our prescriptions closely, dissipating much of the benefit.[30]

Conclusion

Successful bridging of the barriers from evidence to decision making will not ensure that the patient will receive optimal treatment as there are many other factors that might prevail, notably in these days underfunding of health services and maldistribution of resources. Nevertheless, incorporating current best evidence into clinical decisions promises to decrease the traditional delay between evidence generation and application, and to increase the proportion of patients for whom current best treatment is offered. Quick access to accurate summaries of best evidence is rapidly improving at present. Means for creating evidence-based clinical policy and applying this policy judiciously and conscientiously are under development, with this final frontier being advanced by current health services and information research.

References

1 Sackett DL, Rosenberg WMC, Gray JAM, Haynes RB. Evidence based medicine: what it is and what it isn't. *BMJ* 1996;**312**:71–2.
2 Mair F, Crowley T, Bundred P. Prevalence, aetiology, and management of heart failure in general practice. *Br J Gen Pract* 1996;**46**:77–9.
3 Mashru M, Lant A. Interpractice audit of diagnosis and management of hypertension in primary care: educational intervention and review of medical records. *BMJ* 1997;**314**:942–6.
4 Sudlow M, Thomson R, Kenny RA, Rodgers H. A community survey of patients with atrial fibrillation: associated disabilities and treatment preferences. *Br J Gen Pract* 1998;**48**:1775–8.
5 Antman EM, Lau J, Kupelnick B, Mosteller F, Chalmers TC. A comparison of results of meta-analyses of randomized control trials and recommendations of experts. *JAMA* 1992;**268**:240–8.
6 Michaud C, Murray CJL. Resources for health research and development in 1992: a global overview. Annex 5 in: *Investing in health research and development*. Report of the Ad Hoc Committee on Health Research Relating to Future Intervention Options. Geneva: World Health Organization, 1996.
7 Haynes RB. Loose connections between peer-reviewed clinical journals and clinical practice. *Ann Intern Med* 1990;**113**:724–8.
8 Sackett DL, Straus S, Richardson SR, Rosenberg W, Haynes RB. *Evidence-Based Medicine: how to practise and teach EBM.* 2nd edition. London: Churchill Livingstone, 2000.
9 Haynes RB. The origins and aspirations of *ACP Journal Club* [editorial]. *ACP J Club* 1991; Jan-Feb: A18. *Ann Intern Med* 1991;**114**(1).
10 Sackett DL, Haynes RB. On the need for evidence based medicine. *Evidence-Based Med* 1995;**1**:5.
11 *The Cochrane Library*. Oxford: Update Software. Electronic subscription serial.
12 Haynes RB. Advances in evidence-based information resources for clinical practice. *J Pharmaceut Care Pain Sympt Contrl* 1999;**7**:35–49.
13 Hunt DL, Haynes RB, Hanna SE, Smith K. Effects of computer-based clinical decision support systems on physician performance and patient outcomes: a systematic review. *JAMA* 1998;**280**:1339–46.
14 Gray JAM, Haynes RB, Sackett DL, Cook DJ, Guyatt GH. Transferring evidence from health care research into medical practice: 3. Developing evidence based clinical policy. *Evidence-Based Med* 1997;**2**:36–8.
15 Krahn M, Naylor CD, Basinski AS, Detsky AS. Comparison of an aggressive (US) and a less aggressive (Canadian) policy for cholesterol screening and treatment. *Ann Intern Med* 1991;**115**:248–55.
16 Carter A. Background to the "guidelines for guidelines" series. *Can Med Assoc J* 1993;**148**:383.
17 Davis DA, Thomson MA, Oxman AD, Haynes RB. Changing physician performance: a systematic review of the effect of educational strategies. *JAMA* 1995;**274**:700–5.

18 Karuza J, Calkins E, Feather J *et al*. Enhancing physician adoption of practice guidelines. Dissemination of influenza vaccination guideline using a small-group consensus process. *Arch Intern Med* 1995;**155**:625–32.

19 Ketley D, Woods KL. Impact of clinical trials on clinical practice: example of thrombolysis for acute myocardial infarction. *Lancet* 1993;**342**:891–4.

20 Cucherat M, Bonnefoy E, Tremeau G. Primary angioplasty versus intravenous thrombolysis for acute myocardial infarction (Cochrane Review). In: *The Cochrane Library*, Issue 2, 2000. Oxford: Update Software.

21 Grilli R, Lomas J. Evaluating the message: the relationship between compliance rate and the subject of a practice guideline. *Med Care* 1994;**132**:202–13.

22 Aszkenasy OM, Dawson D, Gill M, Haines A, Patterson DLIT. Audit of direct access cardiac investigations: experience in an inner London health district. *J Roy Soc Med* 1994;**87**:588–90.

23 Sutton M. Personal paper: how to get the best health outcome for a given amount of money. *BMJ* 1997;**315**:47–9.

24 Pharoalt PD, Hollingworth W. Cost-effectiveness of lowering cholesterol concentration with statins in patients with and without pre-existing coronary heart disease: life table method applied to health authority population. *BMJ* 1996;**312**:1443–8.

25 European Carotid Surgery Trialists' Collaborative Group. MRC European Carotid Surgery Trial: interim results for symptomatic patients with severe (70–99%) or with mild (0–29%) carotid stenosis. *Lancet* 1991;**337**:1235–43.

26 Stewart M. Studies of health outcomes and patient-centred communication. In: Stewart M, Brown JB, Weston WW, McWhinney IR, McWilliam CL, Freeman TR, eds. *Patient-centred medicine*. California: Sage Publications, 1995.

27 Stocking B. Implementing the findings of effective care in pregnancy and childbirth. *Milbank Q* 1993;**71**:497–522.

28 Murray E, Davis H, See Tai S, Coulter A, Gray A, Haines A. Randomised controlled trial of an interactive multimedia decision aid in hormone replacement therapy. *BMJ* 2001; in press.

29 Murray E, Davis H, See Tai S, Coulter A, Gray A, Haines A. Randomised controlled trial of an interactive multimedia decision aid in benign prostatic hypertrophy. *BMJ* 2001; in press.

30 Haynes RB, Montague P, Oliver T, McKibbon KA, Brouwers MC, Kanani R. Interventions for helping patients to follow prescriptions for medications (Cochrane Review). In: *The Cochrane Library*, Issue 3, 1999. Oxford: Update Software.

11 Decision support systems and clinical innovation

JEREMY C WYATT AND PAUL TAYLOR

Key messages

- Clinical decision support systems are defined and examples given.
- The effectiveness of such systems is considered in terms of barriers to change.
- The knowledge base for decision support systems can be prepared from primary sources or from evidence-based published guidelines.
- Careful consideration must be given to the way in which such systems are integrated into clinical practice.

Introduction

Consider the following scenarios.

- A nurse working in a call centre takes a call from a client. Her computer guides her through a series of questions that establish the most appropriate course of action given the client's symptoms.
- A radiologist interpreting mammograms glances from the film to a digital image on which a computer has indicated areas showing potential abnormalities.
- A member of the public, concerned about his health, accesses a web site, fills in a form with details of his blood pressure and his general health status and, a few seconds later, is given an estimate of his risk of a heart attack.
- A physician working in an anti-coagulant clinic uses a computer model to revise her patient's warfarin dose.

In each of the above scenarios the users have different roles and are making different decisions. What they have in common is that in each a computer is used to assist in making the decision. The systems described are not research projects, they are already in routine use in clinical settings. The decision support systems used by NHS Direct will be involved in

12 million patient episodes in 2001.[1] The R2 Image Checker 2000, already in widespread use in the USA, is currently being evaluated by the NHS Health Technology Assessment programme as a tool for use in breast screening.[2] Cardiac risk calculators are available on numerous web sites, accessible by the general public.[3] The warfarin advisor has been running in the Whittington Hospital since 1992.[4]

These are just a few examples of the variety of clinical decision support systems now available. In each case a computer program embodying knowledge about medicine is used, in combination with information about the patient, to provide advice. This chapter is not, primarily, intended as an introduction to clinical decision support systems nor as a review of research in the field. Rather it is an attempt to explore some specific questions relevant to the themes of the volume. How do the developers of decision support systems obtain the knowledge on which their systems depend? Is it derived from evidence? And if it can be derived from evidence, what is the potential of decision support systems as a way of getting research findings into practice?

First we explain in a little more depth what is meant by the term "clinical decision support system".

Clinical decision support systems

Doctors need to keep abreast of a vast amount of medical knowledge. Smith, reviewing doctors' information needs, concluded that at least one question arises in every doctor-patient consultation and noted that most of these questions seem to go unanswered.[5] Where an answer was sought, the most common course of action is to ask another doctor. The difficulty here is that the doctor being asked the question may not be any more knowledgeable than the doctor seeking an answer. The sources which at the moment are most likely to provide up-to-date and accurate information are, however, too time-consuming and expensive to be used by doctors in the course of their clinical routine: a British study of medical library use found that only 13% of clinicians' requests and searches were carried out solely for patient care.[6] Clinical decision support systems have been developed in an attempt to make available to clinicians, in time to influence decisions, small amounts of knowledge relevant to the patient and the current dilemma. They save the clinician from the need to formulate and carry out a search for medical knowledge, and are usually able not only to provide, but also to explain, advice.

A definition of decision support systems

A clinical decision support system (DSS) is a computer system designed to help health professionals make decisions. In a sense any system which deals

124

with clinical data or medical knowledge is intended to support decisions. In practice, however, the term DSS is usually applied only to systems which help clinicians apply knowledge in particular cases. The definition of the term usually excludes electronic textbooks, hypertext, and text databases which require the user to search for information and do not synthesise search results into a report which applies specifically to a particular patient. Also excluded is educational software, which is designed to enhance a clinician's knowledge, not to assist with specific decisions. Finally, because they do not contain medical knowledge or give advice, computer systems which acquire, process, or communicate patient data are also excluded.

Decision support systems, also called decision aids, consist of a store of medical knowledge, or knowledge base, and a "reasoner" – a computer program which uses patient data to select, display, or apply relevant facts from this knowledge store (Figure 11.1). To obtain advice or information from a DSS, it must be provided with patient data such as the age, clinical findings, diagnosis, current medication, test results, etc. Such data may be entered directly by the clinician or obtained from an electronic patient record or clinical data system.

The term "decision support system" reflects an evolution in thinking about the possible role for computers in decision making, so that they are viewed as having a supporting role: they aim to improve human decision making without replacing human judgement. Their role is analogous to that of an assistant who, given patient data, finds the relevant pages in a

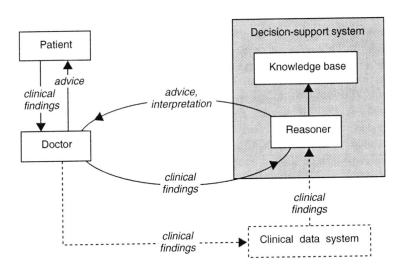

Figure 11.1 A generic model for a decision support system.

125

textbook (the printed counterpart of the knowledge base) and highlights only the material which applies to this patient on this occasion.

Two examples of clinical decision support systems

One of the best known clinical decision support systems is the Quick Medical Reference (QMR) system, which was based on the Internist-1 research project and is now distributed commercially.[7] The system contains a large number of facts about diseases and the clinical findings used in their diagnosis. The user enters clinical findings describing the patient's case. These are used by the system to generate hypotheses. The system gives each hypothesis a score based on the number of findings that would be explained by the hypothesis, the number of findings that it fails to explain and the number of other findings that would have been expected, but which are absent. The user then enters further findings and test results in pursuit of different diagnostic strategies, such as ruling out alternatives or increasing the evidence for the favoured hypothesis.

The knowledge store in QMR contains two sets of facts linking findings and diseases. One records the sensitivity of the finding – the extent to which a finding is suggestive of the disease, the other its positive predictive value – the strength of the expectation that the finding would be present if the patient had the disease. Each is given a rating on a scale of 0–6 or 1–5. The reasoner is the algorithm that uses the ratings to derive a score for each hypothesis and generates the hypothesis set.

The success of the system is critically dependent on the accuracy and completeness of the ratings making up the knowledge base. The procedure followed in developing, extending and updating the system is, therefore, perhaps as interesting as the system itself. The process is organised around the notion of a disease profile, a list of 25 to 250 findings associated with the disease. The knowledge base is extended through the addition of new disease profiles. The creation of a profile involves, first, a search of the relevant textbooks and research literature and next consultation with relevant experts. The results are then reviewed by the QMR project team and tested with "classic" cases.

The knowledge store is therefore based on an expert filtering of the available medical evidence, which suggests that the system could play a role in assisting in the dissemination of new diagnostic evidence. There are problems though. As Antman et al. have shown, textbooks may not be up-to-date.[8] The disease prevalences and even definitions may not apply outside the US. The process of developing and revising profiles is time-consuming and versions of the software can get out of date. It is therefore worth contrasting this kind of decision support system with ones that can be built much more quickly, taking advantage of work that is already being done in systematically collecting and synthesising medical evidence.

One of the first accounts of such a system is the Regenstrief Medical Record system.[9] This system provided decision support based on textual alerts or recommendations developed from management strategies described in the medical literature. For example:

If treatment includes cardiac glycoside and last premature ventricular systoles/minute >2 then recommend "Consider cardiac glycoside as cause of arrhythmia"

These recommendations, termed protocols by McDonald, were incorporated into computer systems that stored the patient's laboratory, medication and vital signs data. When the data matched the events described in a protocol, the associated recommendation was printed out for the doctor. The availability of the recommendations dramatically increased the frequency with which doctors responded to target events, from 22% to 51%.

There are a number of important lessons to be learnt in comparing QMR and the Regenstrief system. The conventional way of using QMR is to access it in the library or on one's own PC. It is therefore rarely used during a patient consultation and many users value it primarily as an educational tool. The McDonald system, in contrast, was integrated into the process of care using pre-printed paper "encounter forms" for the doctor to use during the consultation which carried the computer's recommendations. The reasoner in QMR attempts to emulate diagnostic strategies, its counterpart in the Regenstrief system simply tested to see if events on the record matched those linked to recommendations in the protocols. The knowledge store in QMR requires a laborious process of knowledge elicitation, refinement and engineering; its counterpart is simply the computerisation of the kind of guidelines that are already an important part of clinical practice. These differences have clear implications for the role of DSS as agents for getting research findings into practice. Before addressing these, we give a slightly fuller account of the variety of DSS now in use.

Different kinds of decision support system

Early examples of DSS were developed to help in the diagnosis of patients with acute abdominal pain[10] or the selection of appropriate antibiotic therapies.[11] More recently, systems have been developed to assist in the diagnosis of congenital heart problems,[12] GP prescribing[13] the interpretation of ECG signals[14] and radiological investigations,[15] and to assess prognosis in intensive care units.[16] The range and variety of work in clinical DSS is now such that it would be inappropriate to attempt a complete summary here; interested readers are referred to several short accessible reviews [see for example[17-19]]. It may be useful, however, to provide a short explanation of the differences between the various kinds of

Table 11.1 Some different kinds of decision support system.

Kind of decision support system	Knowledge base contents	Knowledge base origin	Reasoning method
Bayesian model (causal probabilistic network)	Prior and conditional probabilities; causal model	Training data; human expert's causal model	Bayesian probability calculations
Prognostic rule or model	Coefficients of regression formulae	Training data	Calculation of score or probability
Neural network	Node thresholds, strengths of links between nodes	Training data	"Black box" variant of statistical methods
Reminder or alerting system (guideline-based system)	Discrete IF... THEN rules	Practice guideline, human expert, or committee	Conventional programming techniques
Knowledge-based system (expert system)	Facts, rules, semantic networks, frames; uncertainty metrics	Human experts; rules "induced" from training examples	Logic, artificial intelligence techniques

DSS. Systems have been developed using many different techniques for representing medical knowledge, each of which is associated with an appropriate reasoning method. The most common approaches are summarised in Table 11.1. The different approaches vary in the extent to which the knowledge is derived by the system from data – as in neural networks, Bayesian systems and prognostic models – or explicitly represented by the knowledge base author. The difficulty with systems of the former type is first that they are vulnerable to anomalies in the data set on which they were trained, and second that they often have only a limited capacity to explain the advice they provide.

When are decision support systems effective?

A recent study assessed the impact of QMR and one of its competitors, ILIAD, on the performance of 216 US doctors.[20] The study used a set of difficult case scenarios based on real patients. The authors assessed the quality of each doctor's diagnostic reasoning before and after a session using one of the decision support systems. Overall, the correct diagnosis appeared on 40% of doctors' differential diagnosis lists pre DSS and 45% post DSS – an 11% relative increase in diagnostic accuracy. In 12% of cases, the DSS led to the doctor adding the correct diagnosis to their list but in 6% it caused them to drop it, giving a net overall gain of 6%. The net gain was largest for students (9%) and smallest for faculty (3%). QMR produced a net gain of 8%, twice that of the ILIAD system (4·1%).

The authors conclude that the DSS were effective in influencing decision making. However, it is worth noting the caveats. ILIAD was less effective than QMR: if one system is effective it does not show that all systems will be. The impact on students was much greater than the impact on faculty. Worryingly, on 6% of occasions the DSS caused doctors to incorrectly override their own decisions.

A more clinically relevant test of DSS is to examine how often they lead to more appropriate clinical actions and patient outcomes. Hunt systematically reviewed 68 randomised trials of DSS from 1974 to 1997.[21] Of the 65 randomised clinical trials (RCT) in which clinical performance was studied, 43 (66%) showed an improvement. Six (43%) of the 14 studies of patient outcomes showed improvement. Most interesting, however, was the way in which the percentage of studies showing improved actions varied according to the behaviour targeted (Table 11.2).

Table 11.2   Changes in physician performance due to the use of computerised DSS.[21]

Behaviour	Total no. of studies	Studies showing improvement
Diagnosis	5	1 (20%)
Drug dosing	15	9 (60%)
Active clinical care	26	19 (73%)
Preventive care	19	14 (74%)

This shows that the typical complex diagnostic DSS is rarely effective, perhaps because routine clinical practice poses few diagnostic challenges, doctors already excel at diagnosis, or rarely take account of the opinion of a diagnostic DSS.[22] However, the simple reminder systems that advise on active or preventive care frequently lead to improved actions.[9]

It seems clear that decision support systems can improve clinical performance and patient outcome. Equally, it is apparent that many projects end in failure. Some of those in the field have discussed the causes of this failure and proposed a variety of explanations.[22,23,24] Two of the arguments which have been advanced will be picked up in the next section: first, that greater attention should be paid to using rigorous evidence to inform decision support systems and second that the use of guidelines and protocols may provide the most appropriate application for DSS.

Basing decision support systems on evidence

The advice given by a clinical decision support system is based on its computerised knowledge store. The knowledge in decision support systems has rarely been based explicitly on research findings.[22] Constructing this "knowledge base" involves collecting and representing an appropriate set of facts. This process can start by collecting and analysing clinical data, extracting facts from the literature or eliciting them from clinical experts. The latter approach is perhaps the least well grounded in evidence and yet is the most common, as the original impetus for much work in clinical DSS came from artificial intelligence, where the aim was to represent the wisdom of an expert or a group of experts.[11,13] The nature of this paradigm – the "expert system" – has changed, largely through the observation that systems must be designed to work in collaboration with the decision maker, rather than behave like a Greek oracle which elicits information and responds with a preferred solution.[25] The idea that eliciting information from an experienced expert is an acceptable source for a knowledge base has also been questioned,[14,22] but the practice is still widespread.

One notable example of a system that was based on critically appraised research findings is PREOP, a program to help the preoperative work-up of high-risk patients.[26] PREOP elicited input from the user – an internal medical trainee – about the patient and gave advice about drugs and anaesthetic interactions as well as an indication of cardiac risk. The knowledge base consisted of facts systematically extracted from journal articles and books, abstracts of which were available in the system. The authors attempted to practise evidenced-based knowledge base development, but admitted to having had to balance rigour with feasibility. This means that they were obliged to include facts based on lower grade evidence. The criteria used to grade evidence are shown in Table 11.3. Each fact was graded by the strength of evidence, and the best available evidence was presented first.

An alternative to basing the knowledge on findings in the literature or the opinions of experts is primary research carried out specifically to establish the DSS knowledge base. The de Dombal system for the differential diagnosis of acute abdominal pain is the classical example of this.[10] Patient data and gold standard diagnoses were collected over many years to calculate the prior probability of each of the main diseases causing abdominal pain and the conditional probability of symptom S in disease D. Bayes' Theorem was then used to compute the most likely diagnosis from a new patient's symptoms. This relatively simple system assumed that each patient suffered from only one disease and that clinical findings occurred independently. In more recent systems the dependencies between different findings and diseases are represented in a Bayesian network and probabilities associated with each link are obtained from the literature or an expert's subjective judgement, and are then revised in the light of data collected during use of the system. Such systems are thus primed with the available primary or secondary evidence but can continue to "learn" as they are used. Other forms of reasoning for DSS based on primary data such as neural networks are available, but their lack of an explicit knowledge

130

Table 11.3 Criteria used to grade evidence for studies of treatment, prevention, or rehabilitation in PREOP.[26]

Grade	Definition
I	a) random assignment b) control group c) 80% follow-up d) demonstration of a statistically significant difference in at least one important clinical outcome (for example, survival or major morbidity) OR lack of demonstration of a statistically significant difference in an important outcome where power exceeds 80% to detect a clinically important difference
II	As Ia but missing any or all of b, c, or d
III	Non-randomised trial with contemporaneous controls selected by a systematic method
IV	Case series with historical or literature controls OR before-after study OR case series without controls (each should have 10 patients or more)
V	Case report (<10 patients)
VI	Non-clinical study (animal or laboratory tissues, etc.)
VII	None of above (author's unreferenced opinion, experience)

representation and difficulty in inspecting the knowledge base and generating explanations has led to doubts about the use of such "black box" systems to aid clinical decisions.[27]

One response of DSS developers to the problems of building a knowledge base themselves using the primary literature, experts or by carrying out their own studies, is to develop systems which represent one or more evidence-based published guidelines. In effect, the system developer places the responsibility for knowledge base content onto the guideline authors. Such systems are described below.

Guideline-based decision support systems

The idea of a guideline-based DSS is that it will automatically apply the recommendations from an evidence-based guideline to screen patients before or during the clinical encounter for potential preventive care opportunities, changes to drug or test orders, possible hazards or other conditions, freeing the clinician to focus on broader issues. To achieve this, guideline-based DSSs need access to extensive coded patient data, as few clinicians will wish to enter such structured data themselves. This means that guideline based DSSs are best applied in organisations where much clinical data is already computerised in coded form (not as scanned or dictated text), which can be reliably linked to the patient in question using a single identifier.[28] Such coded data can be obtained from a pharmacy information system (to generate a list of past and current prescribed drugs), an order communication system (to obtain laboratory and imaging results and orders pending) and other parts of an electronic patient record (to provide a coded list of clinical problems, allergies etc.). In addition, for the guideline-based DSS to alter what doctors do and patient outcomes, as they see the patient and make their decisions the clinician must either use a networked computer or a structured, computer-generated paper encounter form carrying DSS recommendations.

Some US hospitals have evolved such fully integrated clinical information systems[9,28,29,30] but there are few if any in the UK. Thus, the first challenge with implementing guideline-based DSS is not developing the DSS itself but finding a site with the essential infrastructure – coded patient data, universal patient identifiers and point-of-care information systems.

The DSS enthusiast might assume that the UK electronic patient record programme[31] and the plethora of practice guidelines now means that such systems will soon be implemented, but success means passing at least 10 challenging stages:

1 Get local agreement for the innovation process and identify a suitable up-to-date, evidence-based guideline
2 Examine the individual and organisational barriers to change using the PRECEDE model[32] and assess the viability of DSS reminders as a method for overcoming these barriers. Sometimes, other innovation methods may be more appropriate
3 Tailor the chosen guideline and its recommendations to local circumstances,[32] taking account of the local barriers, case mix, resources, clinical setting, preferences etc.
4 Identify the relevant recommendations in the guideline and the significant entities they rely on, such as items of patient data to be collected, normal ranges for laboratory tests and actions such as drug prescribing or test ordering
5 Ensure that all local information systems such as electronic patient record, laboratory and prescribing systems share common codes or names for the significant entities used in the guideline such as each item of patient data, drug or test to be carried out
6 Ensure that each significant entity in the guideline can be reliably translated in terms of the common codes used in local information systems (for example the guideline may exclude patients with "recent prior antibiotic use" – how will such patients be identified?)
7 Model relevant guideline recommendations as condition-action statements for the DSS knowledge base, taking account of the need to translate the significant named entities to the local codes for data and actions
8 Test and debug the DSS rules with recent patient data and check that the advice is appropriate

9   Release the new rules and monitor their impact on clinical decisions, actions and patient outcomes

10   Revise as necessary.

Capturing and representing the condition-action statements in the knowledge base is thus only one part of this whole process, but a number of projects have focused on this. One has developed a language, PROforma, for expressing guidelines and a graphical knowledge base editor tool to allow relatively inexperienced users to enter guideline knowledge in this form.[33] One potential benefit of such tools is that they could allow a trained clinician to help keep such a guideline-based DSS up to date.

There is also the potential for national guideline authors to use such tools instead of word processors during the primary guideline development process, to help them identify and eliminate the inevitable inconsistencies and gaps in their guideline. There is an international proposal for a Guideline Interchange Format and associated databases to support the exchange of guidelines[34] with the developers of guideline authoring and

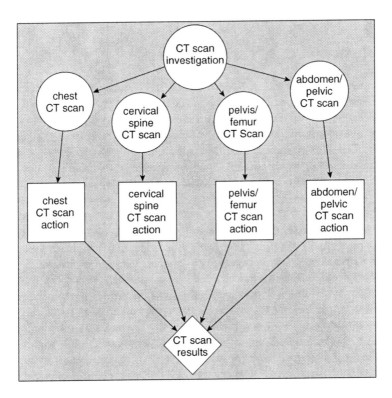

Figure 11.2 A fragment of a clinical guideline represented in the graphical editor used with PROforma.

133

"enactment" tools seeking to converge their own representations. However, national guidelines often need tailoring to fit local circumstances even in the same country, while there are often marked differences between evidence-based guidelines for the same condition from different countries, reflecting valid differences of opinion and available resources. It would therefore be a mistake to disseminate guideline knowledge bases unchanged to local health organisations without allowing them to inspect and modify certain portions. Deciding which portions can be safely altered, and by how much, remains a key challenge.

As examples of such systems, Safran *et al.* described a controlled trial of a computer-based patient record system which generated guideline-derived messages to alert clinicians to events likely to occur in HIV patients.[29] They found greatly reduced response times to the events when alerts were issued compared to response times when no alert was issued. Pestonik *et al.* carried out a study of the use of DSS with local clinician-derived guidelines for antibiotic therapy.[30] They found antibiotic use was improved, costs were reduced, and the emergence of antibiotic-resistant pathogens was stabilised.

Conclusions

Forty years of research into computer-based medical decision support systems since the first paper[35] have led to the publication of thousands of papers reporting apparently successful systems, but very few of these were ever implemented in clinical settings and even fewer describe rigorous studies. The 793 citations identified in an early systematic review of DSS by Johnston *et al.* included only 28 controlled trials, of which 21 were, to some degree, methodologically flawed.[36] Clearly, there is considerable scope for system developers to improve the rigour with which they evaluate their technology.[37] Even then, 18 out of the 28 trials demonstrated clear benefits from the use of these systems, but the field has had relatively little impact on clinical practice. For some the lack of diffusion of these tools is due to resistance by medical professionals, for others the tools fail to capture the essence of human practice. It seems that both DSS tools and clinical practice need to develop together and transform each other, as has happened in the case of telephone triage systems.[38]

Proponents of evidence-based practice argue for an increased formalisation of medicine and the adoption of formal skills and tools to guide clinical practice. Inserting a formal tool such as a computer system – or a guideline – into a clinical setting inevitably alters the setting, through the establishment or reinforcement of bureaucratic hierarchies, increased structuring of medical work (for example, through use of standard data collection forms), and a concentration on data items which can be gathered reliably and unequivocally, to the exclusion of useful but unstructured information such as details of a patient's home life. We need, therefore, to understand the consequences of adopting such tools in clinical settings.

Berg argues that we need to step outside the discipline of the system designer and understand the social, material, and organisational aspects of medical work.[38] The process of designing a new tool also implies constructing a new niche, not shaping the tool to fit a pre-existing niche. Poor design and a failure to consider the practicalities and barriers to change in clinical settings have hindered the take-up of decision support systems, but such systems could never be designed to fit seamlessly into existing ways of working since their use inevitably changes practice. And they do so in ways which have drawbacks as well as benefits. The challenge, as stated by Berg, is to search for ways in which decision support systems can become "familiar yet never totally transparent, powerful yet fragile agents of change". It seems likely that DSS will provide not just an effective technology to facilitate the implementation of research findings and clinical innovation, but may also help us to understand how some of the barriers to innovation arise and may be overcome.

Davis *et al.* compared the effectiveness of DSS with other ways of changing clinical practice, in a review of 101 randomised trials of innovation methods, again checking how many led to improved clinical practice, with the results shown in Table 11.4.[39]

Reminder (largely decision support) systems were more effective at improving clinical actions than continuing education, audit and feedback, mailed educational materials or patient mediated interventions, but less effective than methods based on outreach or opinion leaders. It should be noted that these results came from a wide range of settings and perhaps the DSS were used with clinical practices that were easier to alter. The only rigorous way to determine if a DSS is more effective than another innovation method is to conduct a comparison within the same study. However, there are as yet very few within-study comparisons.

The further development of evidence-based practice will result in the increasing use of guidelines based on sound evidence. This will be facilitated

Table 11.4 Results of randomised trials of innovation methods for improving clinical practice.

Innovation	Success rate
Formal continuing education course	1/7 (14%)
Mailed educational materials	4/11 (36%)
Audit and feedback	10/24 (42%)
Patient mediated (for example leaflets)	7/9 (78%)
Reminders to clinicians (i.e. DSS)	22/26 (85%)
Outreach visits	7/7 (100%)
Opinion leaders	3/3 (100%)

by, and provide an application for, decision support systems. The role of DSS in evidence-based practice is not, however, restricted to systems which assist in guideline-directed care. DSS are also being developed to assist in the design of randomised controlled trials[40] and to support the screening, recruitment and data collection from patients enrolled in trials, to help us discover the evidence on which future patient management and policy decisions are based.[41]

References

1 Munro J, Nicholl J, O'Cathain A, Knowles E. Impact of NHS Direct on demand for immediate care: observational study. *BMJ* 2000;**321**:150–3.
2 Taylor P. Computer aided detection *Breast Cancer Res* 2000;**2**:S11.
3 International Task Force for Prevention of Coronary Heart Disease Procam Risk Calculator http://www.chd-taskforce.de/calculator/calculator.htm (accessed 14 November 2000).
4 Vadher B, Patterson DLH, Leaning M. Evaluation of a decision support system for initiation and control of oral anticoagulation in a randomised trial. *BMJ* 1997;**314**:1252–6.
5 Smith R. What clinical information do doctors need? *BMJ* 1996;**313**:1062–8.
6 Urquart C, Hepworth J. The value of information supplied to clinicians by health libraries: devising an outcomes-based assessment of the contribution of libraries to clinical decision making. *Health Libr Rev* 1995;**12**:201–15.
7 Miller RA, Pople HE, Myers J. Internist-I: an experimental computer-based diagnostic consultant for general internal medicine. *N Engl J Med* 1982;**307**:468–76.
8 Antman E, Lau J, Kupelnick B *et al.* A comparison of the results of meta-analysis of randomised controlled trials and recommendations of clinical experts. *JAMA* 1992;**268**:240–8.
9 McDonald CJ. Protocol-based computer reminders, the quality of care and the non-perfectability of man. *N Engl J Med* 1976;**295**:1351–5.
10 De Dombal FT, Leaper DJ, Staniland JR *et al.* Computer-aided diagnosis of acute abdominal pain. *BMJ* 1972;**2**:9–13.
11 Shortliffe E. *Computer-based medical consultations: MYCIN.* Artificial Intelligence Series. New York: Elsevier Computer Science Library, 1976.
12 Franklin RC, Spiegelhalter DJ, Macartney FJ, Bull K. Evaluation of a diagnostic algorithm for heart disease in neonates. *BMJ* 1991;**302**:935–9.
13 Walton RT, Gierl C, Yudkin P *et al.* Evaluation of computer support for prescribing (CAPSULE) using simulated cases. *BMJ* 1997;**315**:791–5.
14 Wyatt J. Promoting routine use of medical knowledge systems: lessons from computerised ECG interpreters. In: Barahona P, Christensen JP, eds. *Knowledge and decisions in health telematics.* Amsterdam: IOS Press, 1994.
15 Taylor P, Fox J, Todd-Pokropek A. The Development and Evaluation of CADMIUM: a prototype system to assist in the interpretation of mammograms. *Medical Image Analysis* 1999;**3**:321–37.
16 Knaus WA, Wagner DP, Lynn J. Short-term mortality predictions for critically ill, hospitalised adults: science and ethics. *Science* 1991;**254**:389–94.
17 Miller RA. Medical diagnostic decision support systems – past, present, and future. *J Am Med Inform Assoc* 1994;**1**:8–27.
18 Van Bemmel J and Musen M (eds.) *The Handbook of Medical Informatics.* Heidelberg: Springer-Verlag 1997.
19 Wyatt JC. Knowledge for the clinician 9. Decision support systems. *JRSM* 2000;**93**:629–33.
20 Friedman CP, Elstein AS, Wolf FM *et al.* Enhancements of clinicians' diagnostic reasoning by computer based consultation. *JAMA* 1999;**282**:1851–6.
21 Hunt DL, Haynes RB, Hanna SE, Smith K. Effects of computer-based clinical decision support systems on physician performance and patient outcomes: a systematic review. *JAMA* 1998;**280**:1339–46.

22 Heathfield H, Wyatt J. Philosophies for the design and development of clinical decision support systems. *Methods Inf Med* 1993;**32**:1–9.
23 Coiera E. Question the assumptions. In: Barahona P, Christensen JP, eds. *Knowledge and decisions in health telematics*. Amsterdam: IOS Press, 1994.
24 Van der Lei J. Computer-based decision support: the unfulfilled promise. In: Barahona P, Christensen JP, eds. *Knowledge and decisions in health telematics*. Amsterdam: IOS Press, 1994.
25 Miller RA, Masarie FE. The demise of the Greek oracle model for medical diagnostic systems. *Methods Inf Med* 1990;**29**:1–3.
26 Holbrook A, Langton K, Haynes RB *et al.* PREOP: development of an evidence-based expert system to assist with pre-operative assessments. In: Clayton P, ed. *Proceedings of the 15th Symposium on Computer Applications in Medical Care*. New York: McGraw Hill, Inc., 1991.
27 Wyatt J. Nervous about artificial neural networks? *Lancet* 1995;**346**:1175–7 (editorial).
28 Bleich HL, Beckley RF, Horowitz GL *et al.* Clinical computing in a teaching hospital. *N Engl J Med* 1985;**312**:756–64.
29 Safran C, Rind DM, Davis RB *et al.* Guidelines for management of HIV infection with computer-based patient records. *Lancet* 1995;**346**:341–6.
30 Pestotnik SL, Classen DC, Evans RS, Burke JP. Implementing antibiotic practice guidelines through computer-assisted decision support: clinical and financial outcomes. *Ann Intern Med* 1996;**124**:884–90.
31 NHS Executive, *Information for Health*. London: HMSO, 1998.
32 Wyatt JC. Knowledge for the clinician 3. Practice guidelines and other support for clinical innovation. *J R Soc Med* 2000;**93**:299–304.
33 Fox J, Johns N, Rahmanzadeh A, Thompson R. ProForma: a general technology for clinical decision support systems. *Comput Methods Programs Biomed* 1997;**54**:59–67.
34 Ohno-Machado L, Gennari JH, Murphy SN *et al.* The Guideline Interchange Format: a model for representing guidelines. *J Am Med Inform Assoc* 1998;**5**:357–72.
35 Hollingsworth TH. Using an electronic computer in a problem of medical diagnosis. *J Roy Stat Soc A* 1959;**122**:221–31.
36 Johnston ME, Langton KB, Hayes B, Mathieu A. Effects of computer-based clinical decision support systems on clinician performance and patient outcome. *Ann Intern Med* 1994;**120**:135–42.
37 Friedman CP, Wyatt JC. *Evaluation methods in medical informatics*. New York: Springer Verlag, 1998.
38 Berg M. *Rationalizing medical work*. Cambridge, Massachusetts: MIT Press, 1997.
39 Davis DA, Thomson MA, Oxman AD, Haynes RB. A systematic review of the effect of continuing medical education strategies. *JAMA* 1995;**274**:700–5.
40 Wyatt JC, Altman DG, Heathfield HA, Pantin CF. Development of Design-a-Trial, a knowledge-based critiquing system for authors of clinical trial protocols. *Comput Methods Programs Biomed* 1994;**43**:283–91.
41 Carlson RW, Tu SW, Lane NM *et al.* Computer-based screening of patients with HIV/AIDS for clinical trial eligibility. *On-line J Clin Trials* 1995; Doc. no. 179.

12 Decision analysis and the implementation of research findings

R J LILFORD, S G PAUKER, DAVID BRAUNHOLTZ, AND JIRI CHARD

Key messages

- Currently, research results and other information are usually used in decision making (whether for individual patients or for resource allocation) in a way which is informal, idiosyncratic, and opaque.
- Decision Analysis (DA) is a framework for decision making that is transparent, explicit, and logical.
- DA explicitly incorporates both information (eg, from research) and values attributed to outcomes (eg, by the patient).
- Uncertainty about key parameters (eg, true death rates with and without treatment) is expressed using subjective, Bayesian probabilities.
- A set of 'specimen' DAs, with varying patient characteristics and values, can help busy clinicians deliver evidence-based treatment for individual patients.
- By highlighting where current factual uncertainty could impact strongly on decisions, DA can identify which future research would be most useful.

Introduction

Evidence-based medicine consists of more than just reading the results of research and applying them to patients. This is because patients have particular features which may make them atypical of the "average" patient studied in, for example, a clinical trial.[1] These particularities are of two types:

(1) factors affecting probability, for example, the probability that treatments will have the same (absolute and relative) effects as those measured in the trial

(2) the values (or utilities) which affect how much side-effect a person is prepared to trade off against treatment advantages.

138

For these reasons, it is necessary to particularise from trial results. This is usually done intuitively but decision analysis provides the intellectual framework for an explicit decision making algorithm, the rigor of which can be subject to criticism and improvement. However, it is currently unrealistic (due to time constraints) to do a decision analysis separately for each patient. In the long term, computer programs may enable us to overcome this problem. In the meantime, decision analyses can be done for categories of patient with similar clinical features and personal utilities. The results of such "generic" decision analyses are a sound basis for guidelines. Decision analysis thus provides a rational *interpretative* function to get from evidence to implementation.

Decision analysis is described in detail elsewhere,[2-5] but essentially it involves constructing a flow diagram or decision tree showing the available choices and their possible consequences. The probabilities of the various outcomes (contingent upon treatment options and antecedent events) are then added to the diagram. Lastly, the value of each outcome – its relative desirability or undesirability – is incorporated as a so-called "utility". Given the flow diagram, the probabilities, and the individual utilities, the "best" treatment can be calculated. This is the treatment which maximises expected utility by taking into account the probabilities of the various outcomes and how these are valued. The numerical calculations (once probabilities and values are known) are very easy. We will explain decision analysis with an example.

An example – how does it work in practice?

Megatrials[6] show that clot-busting drugs save lives in suspected myocardial infarction (MI). However, these drugs can cause stroke which may leave the patient severely incapacitated. Also, there is a choice of drugs - the genetically engineered "accelerated" tissue plasminogen activator (tPA) is more effective in preventing death from heart attack than streptokinase (SK), but it has a higher chance of causing a stroke. The risk of causing a stroke does not depend on when treatment is given. However, the probability of preventing death from heart attack does depend on how soon treatment begins after onset of symptoms and on individual risks. Individual risks depend on the probability that the patient has actually had a heart attack and the risk of death given a heart attack. Further complicating the picture, the relative advantage of tPA over SK in preventing cardiac death dissipates after about six hours, and thrombolytic drugs can cause other complications (haemorrhage and anaphylaxis).

So what do we do about all these factors? Kellett and Clarke[7] did a systematic review and then modelled all these variables by decision analysis. We have distilled the probabilities of the main outcomes in Table 12.1 and reproduced a simplified decision diagram in Figure 12.1. "Specimen" utilities

Table 12.1 Probabilities of various events (expressed as percentages) according to therapy, aspirin by itself or with either streptokinase or tPA.

	a (with aspirin)	b (with streptokinase)	c (with tissue plasminogen activator)
P3 = probability of dying of myocardial infarction	11·5	$11·5 \times 0·75 = 8·6$	$8·6 \times 0·8 = 6·9$
P4 = probability of surviving CVA	0·2	0·5	0·7
P5 = probability of dying from CVA	0·2	0·5	0·7
P6 = probability of dying from haemorrhage or anaphylaxis	0	0·2	0·18
P2 = survival without stroke given MI = $1 - (p3 + p4 + p5 + p6)$	88·1	90·2	91·5
P8 = death from another cause sans MI	2·0	2·0	2·0
P9 = survival from stroke sans MI	0	0·4	0·6
P10 = death from stroke sans MI	0	0·4	0·6
P11 = death from complications sans MI	0	0·08	0·06
P7 = intact	98	97·1	96·74

are used for the various outcomes; a value of 1 for healthy survival and 0 for death. About half the victims of stroke in these circumstances will survive, but often with incapacity – the mean utility of post-stroke existence is 0·5.[8] The results of running the base case model (i.e. for a person "typical" of participants in trials of thrombolysis) are shown in Table 12.2. Clearly, there is much expected utility to be gained by giving a clot buster and, moreover, tPA is the drug of choice. Even if we assume a passionate desire to avoid the disability of stroke, giving it a utility of −1 (i.e. a healthy person who would equate a 20% risk of death with a 10% risk of stroke), the above therapies remain optimal (data not shown). However, we get very different results as we move away from the base case. For example, chest pain in a 55-year-old man with a normal ECG is associated with a risk of MI of only 17%, and clot busters stand to lower expected utility in these circumstances. The same man with normal ST but an abnormal T-wave on the ECG has about a 24% risk of MI – thrombolysis is advantageous, but only just, and it would be disadvantageous if he was younger (his risk of dying given a MI would drop to 5% at age 45), if presentation was late (after six hours or so), or if the patient was particularly strongly averse to residual morbidity from stroke.

The model presented here is for teaching purposes and it has been simplified accordingly from the original published work (see below), although not as much as clinicians trying to do it all intuitively. Nevertheless, once the relevant spreadsheet has been set up, it is possible to quickly alter probabilities to take additional factors into account. For example, we may wish

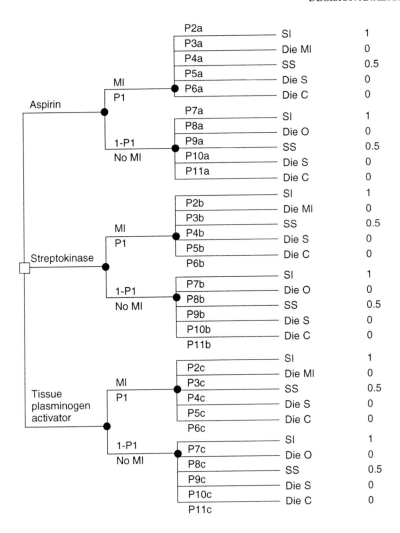

Figure 12.1 Decision tree for the choice of aspirin only versus plus streptokinase versus plus tissue plasminogen activator for the treatment of suspected acute myocardial infarction. The figures on the far right of the diagram are the values. (SI = survive intact; SS = survive stroke; Die S = die of stroke; Die C = die of complications [haemorrhage or anaphalaxis]; Die O = die of another disease masquerading as MI.)

The formulae for expected utilitie s are:

Aspirin P1{(1*P2a) + (0*P3a) + (0.5*P4a) + (0*P5a) + (0*P6a)} +
(1 − P1) {(1*P7a) + (0*P8a) + (0.5*P9a) + (0*P10a) + (0*P11a)}

SK P1{(1*P2b) + (0*P3b) + (0.5*P4b) + (0*P5b) + (0*P6b)} +
(1 − P1) {(1*P7b) + (0*P8b) + (0.5*P9b) + (0*P10b) + (0*P11b)}

tPA P1{(1*P2c) + (0*P3c) + (0.5*P4c) + (0*P5c) + (0*P6c)} +
(1 − P1) {(1*P7c) + (0*P8c) + (0.5*P9c) + (0*P10c) + (0*P11c)}

141

Table 12.2 Relative expected utilities (U) of aspirin only (a) versus plus streptokinase (SK) versus plus accelerated tissue plasminogen activator (tPA) given different probabilities of myocardial infarction (MI) and death given MI (all expressed as percentages). (Relative ranking of utilities as in Figure 12.1. The "base case" is highlighted.)

Probability of MI	Probability of death given MI	% improvement with SK* over a	% improvement with tPA over SK*	USK-Ua	UtPA-Ua	Corollary i.e. Guideline
17	11·5	25	20	−0·00186	−0·00173	At low probabilities of a heart attack, give aspirin only.
17	5·0	25	20	−0·00463	−0·00615	
17	11·5	15	0	−0·00382	−0·0662	
24	11·5	25	20	+0·00017	+0·00152	At moderate probabilities of a heart attack, give clot busters only if presenting in first six hours and if prognosis given MI is in the moderate to severe category (for example over 5%). Use tPA. Benefit is marginal.
24	5·0	25	20	−0·00373	−0·00473	
24	11·5	15	0	−0·00259	−0·00539	
90	**11·5**	**25**	**20**	**+0·01935**	**+0·03207**	At high probabilities of MI, give clot busters and use tPA only if less than six hour history. Even at these high probabilities, the benefits disappear if survival with stroke is given a disutility of −1 and either the prognosis for survival is high (95%) or delay is considerable – data not shown.
90	5·0	25	20	+0·00472	+0·00867	
90	11·5	15	0	+0·00899	+0·00619	

*These figures are dependent on duration of symptoms.
NB. A negative figure indicates that aspirin only is preferable.

to consider the adverse effect of clot busters on patients with dissecting aneurysm. We did this by adding an extra percentage risk of death when clot busters are given to people with no MI. This makes little difference to the base case but now makes clot busters the less favoured option in people with lower (25%) prior risk of heart attack, even in the small group where they were otherwise beneficial. Some people may have a higher risk of stroke, say, because of severe hypertension. When this extra risk crosses a "threshold" of fourfold, thrombolysis is no longer the preferred option, even for the base case. We have not taken into account the likelihood that clot busters administered within six hours protect against congestive heart failure (CHF) – reducing this risk from baseline (about 20%) by perhaps four percentage points (life with CHF is valued, on average, at about 0·9). Also, we have treated the problem as having a fixed time horizon, whereas in reality those with CHF and stroke disability have lower life expectancy than those with uncomplicated MI who in turn have lower life expectancy than survivors of non-MI chest pain. For example, the impact of stroke should include not only a measure of the disutility of each year of disability, but also the reduced expected survival. This can be achieved by calculating and summing expected utilities for each potential remaining year. In other words, a calculation like that in Figure 12.1 is repeated for each future year of life that might be lived. The calculations are different for each year by the probabilities that people in one state (for example, healthy survival following MI) will move to another state (for example, death). This is called a Markov process[9] and can easily be handled on a spreadsheet or specific decision analysis software. In the event, two of these factors (possibility of CHF and flexible time horizon) were taken into account in a masterful decision analysis conducted by Kellett and Clarke[7], and the decision was not "sensitive" to these factors, i.e. the more comprehensive approach gave similar (albeit intellectually more robust) conclusions.

Decision analysis seems the only way to make sense of the complex world of decisions. However, it raises many interesting issues.

- How may probabilities best be derived from the evidence base?
- How may utilities be measured and whose utilities are used?
- Is decision analysis a way of having a debate about general issues in care or is it a way to treat individual patients (or both)?
- How can decision analysis be used to make decisions which affect groups of people?

Probability

Probability lies at the heart of most clinical research; evidence-based practice is practice underpinned by evidence about probabilities. Probability is also fundamental to decision analysis. It is therefore important to understand probability in more detail.

143

Clinicians are most familiar with probability in the form of the predictive value of test results (noting that test is used here to denote any information about a patient, not only results from the laboratory). Take a woman who is pregnant for the first time, whose brother had classic Duchenne dystrophy, diagnosed by elevated creatine kinase (CK) levels, and who died of heart failure. She has no living male relatives on her mother's side of the family, and her mother is also dead. In the absence of any other information and the inability to obtain DNA samples from an affected family member or from her mother, this woman has one chance in three of being a carrier for the disease (this takes account of the fact that a third of all cases of Duchenne dystrophy are new mutations). Typically, in medicine, we do not have just one piece of information about our patient. For example, in the case of the above patient with a genetic history of muscular dystrophy, we may have a serum CK level. Such additional information seldom discriminates perfectly between affected and unaffected individuals, and such is the case with CK.[10] The literature suggests that 70% of carriers will have elevated serum CK levels. Because the normal range is typically defined as the mean plus or minus two standard deviations, 2·5% of normal women (the upper tail) will have elevated serum levels. A simple method for "updating" probabilities according to test results is shown in Table 12.3. A simplified form of Bayes' theorem applies in situations, such as the one at

Table 12.3 Using Bayes' theorem to interpret serum creatine kinase (CK) in a potential Duchenne muscular dystrophy carrier.

Elevated CK

A Diagnosis	B Prior probability	C Conditional probability of elevated CK	D Product (B × C)	E Posterior probability
Carrier	33	70·0	2310·0	93·2%
Not carrier	67	2·5	167·5	6·8%
		Sum =	2477·5	

Normal CK

A Diagnosis	B Prior probability	C Conditional probability of normal CK	D Product (B × C)	E Posterior probability
Carrier	33	30·0	990·0	13·2%
Not carrier	67	97·5	6532·5	86·8%
		Sum =	7522·5	

NB. Upper half of table is for an elevated CK; the lower half is for a normal CK. For each analysis, Column A contains the possible diagnoses, in this case only two, but in general there could be several. Column B contains the prior probability of each diagnosis on a consistent scale (this would be the probability of a woman whose single brother had confirmed Duchenne dystrophy and who had no other known male relatives from her maternal line). Column C contains the conditional probability of the observed result for each diagnosis. Column D contains the product of columns B and C for each diagnosis. Column E contains the revised or posterior probabilities (shown as percentages) and is calculated by dividing each product (in column D) by the sum of the products in column D.

hand, wherein the test can only be positive or negative and a single state or disease (in this example the carrier state) is either present or absent. The ratio of the probability of the observed CK level if the patient is or is not a carrier is known as the likelihood ratio. Given the prior odds (and recalling that odds are simply a ratio of probabilities) and the likelihood ratio for the observed test result, it is easy to calculate the revised (posterior) odds (and hence probability) that the patient is a carrier simply by multiplying the prior odds by the likelihood ratio. For example, in this case the prior odds are 1 : 2 and the likelihood ratio for an elevated CK is 70/2·5 or 28; thus the posterior odds are 14 : 1, corresponding to a probability of 93%. Further, as data are typically acquired sequentially, one test after the next, the techniques of probability revision need to be applied in a stepwise fashion, with the posterior probability calculated from one step becoming the prior for the next. Some care is needed where tests are not providing independent information on disease state, as the magnitude of the appropriate (conditional) likelihood ratio of the second test may be much reduced.

Intervention studies (typically clinical trials) provide probabilities on the effects of treatments. These studies can be analysed to give two kinds of probability: conventional and Bayesian. Conventional (frequentist) statistics give "p" values and confidence limits which are based on the probability of seeing the observed (or a more extreme) result, given a true state of the world. This depends on assumptions about the true underlying state of the world. However, decision analysis (and indeed, "bedside" decisions generally) require not the probability of already observed results given some true underlying state of the world, but rather the (posterior) probabilities of particular differences in the effects, given the observed data.[11] Imagine a trial comparing treatments X and Y has measured a 10 percentage point improvement in survival with Y. A patient, who is similar in relevant characteristics to those in the trial, does not want to know that this observed improvement has only a 2·5% chance of occurring, *if* the treatments are equivalent. She needs to know the probability that improvement in survival with treatment Y compared to treatment X really is (say) 10 or more percentage points. Such probabilities – describing beliefs – are known as Bayesian, and their calculation requires that a prior belief (expressed as a probability distribution) be updated according to the research results obtained. An example showing how this works (without going into the mathematics at all) is shown in Figure 12.2. Bayesian statistics give a probability distribution for the true value of a parameter, such as number needed to treat (NNT) – the number of patients who on average would need to receive a treatment in order for one extra patient to benefit. A clear measure of the uncertainty in our knowledge of a parameter provides a rational basis for decision taking. The relative effects of tissue plasminogen activator (TPA) and streptokinase have been reanalysed along Bayesian lines and the putative advantages of the more expensive therapy

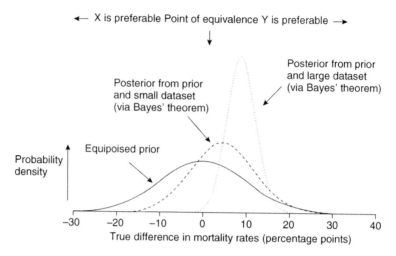

$\longleftarrow$ X is preferable   Point of equivalence   Y is preferable $\longrightarrow$

Figure 12.2 The "prior" distribution of probabilities sums up an individual's beliefs prior to seeing new evidence. Suppose a clinician is equipoised i.e. has no reason to believe treatment X is superior or inferior to treatment Y, both resulting in a mortality rate around 50%. She believes a difference in (true) mortality rate of up to 10% points either way is fairly likely, but that a difference of more than 20% points either way is unlikely. She chooses a normal prior (for convenience - the algebra works out more easily) for the percentage point treatment difference, centred on zero difference, and with a standard deviation (SD) of 10% points. This is actually "equivalent" to the information which would arise from a hypothetical trial with 50 patients and 25 deaths in each arm.

Suppose there is now information from a small trial, with 40 patients in each arm. With treatment Y, 18 patients die, whereas with X, 22 patients die. The observed mortality difference is 10% points. This evidence is combined with the prior belief to produce "posterior" beliefs (which is what her beliefs should now logically be, given the evidence and her prior beliefs). As can be seen above, this posterior is a normal distribution centred a little less than half way between 0 and 10, and with SD somewhat less than that of the prior. The trial evidence has made the clinician's beliefs more precise by adding to her knowledge (reducing the SD), but in fact she remains slightly more influenced by the prior than by the trial. She can calculate posterior probabilities that, for example, treatment Y is superior to X (P=0·73), or that treatment Y is 10% points or more superior to X (P=0·23), etc.

Suppose, on the other hand, there becomes available data from a large trial of 400 patients in each arm, with 180 and 220 patients dying with treatments Y and X respectively. The figure shows that the posterior resulting from combining this with the prior is a much narrower (i.e. more informative) normal distribution centred just below the observed difference of 10% points. Here, the trial is providing a lot more information than the prior. The posterior probability that Y is superior is now 0·996, while the probability that Y is superior by 10% points or more is 0·37.

(TPA) was thereby called into question. Given a reasonably sceptical prior, the results of clinical trials are much less impressive when analysed on Bayesian lines than when analysed by simple p values and confidence intervals.[12,13]

In our example of heart attack we considered two kinds of patient variable. Firstly, there are variables which affect *absolute* but not *relative* treatment effects. Thus people in the 40–49, 50–59, and 60–69 age bands all receive a 25% improvement in mortality with SK, but the absolute gain is greater in the high-risk older group. The second type of patient variable has an influence on *relative* treatment effects. Thus the duration of symptoms affected the efficiency of SK relative to aspirin so that the improvement in mortality reduces from over 25% at less than three hours to no effect at 24 hours. Of course, if trials were infinitely large then we could look up the precise relative treatment effect for any given category of patient. However, even when overall effects are measured precisely in trials, the effects in sub-groups (strata) are typically imprecise. "What to do" – take the overall effect and apply it to the subgroup or use the imprecise measurement made in the sub-groups? For example, the International Study of Infarct Survival (ISIS-II)[6] trial of clot-busting drugs was analysed in sub-groups. Unsurprisingly, this showed a null effect for people who had had their pain for a long time, but unexpectedly also for those born under the star sign Gemini. On what basis can we "believe" one sub-group analysis and not the other? In a Bayesian sub-group analysis we must give our prior beliefs for how the effect in the sub-group may relate to the effect in the remainder.[14,15] We are almost certain that there is little (or no) difference between Geminis and non-Geminis. The observed difference will therefore fail to shift our prior (or shift it very little) and our posterior will remain that Geminis and non-Geminis benefit similarly. Our prior for the difference between patients with prolonged pain and others would (1) be less precise and (2) reflect our belief that those with prolonged pain stand to benefit less than patients with short-duration pain, i.e. from our knowledge of drugs and infarcts, we expect any benefits to be largest if these drugs are administered quickly. In this case the data reinforces our prior belief and enables us to be more precise about how benefit reduces with increasing delay.

Values

The great strength of decision analysis is that it is based not just on probabilities but on how the outcomes are valued. It therefore represents a method for synthesising both the medical facts (probabilities) and the human values which *together* determine the best course of action – that with the maximum expected utility.[16] Decision analysis therefore reconciles "evidence-based medicine" with "preference-based medicine".

Of course, there is an issue here about how these values can best be obtained. At heart, values imply a trade-off – the extent which the disadvantages of one outcome can be offset by the advantages of another. For example, survival with radical surgery is higher than with radiotherapy for patients with cancer of the larynx. However, such surgery obviously limits the ability to speak. There is then a trade-off between survival (maximised by surgery) and the ability to communicate (which is retained to a much better degree with radiotherapy). If a patient would run a 10% chance of dying to avoid loss of the power of speech, then she values life with this impediment at 0·9, on a scale from 1·0 (healthy life) to 0 (death). In the example above, the valuation for life impeded by the effect of stroke was 0·5. The subject of the measurement of human values is a huge one which has been reviewed by many authors.[17–21]

Sensitivity analysis, generic decision analysis, and the individual patient

When consulting an individual, it is important to elicit personal values or at least to get a sense of these. However, it is not essential to redo the analysis for every patient in a busy clinic. Decision analysis may also be done outside the consulting room using a selection of different probability and utility figures within a reasonable range – sensitivity analysis. We used this technique to see how the expected utility of clot-busting drugs may vary by medical and psychological characteristics to produce the guidelines in Table 12.2. The sequence of events forming a decision analysis-based guideline and applying it is shown in Figure 12.3.

Often, short-term outcomes are available from clinical trials but long-term outcomes must be derived, as best they can, from observational studies. Since long-term outcomes are often of greatest importance to patient and payer, these should be "modelled" by decision analysis. For example, modelling was required to extrapolate the results of a trial evaluating short-term effects of different types of angioplasty beyond the information collected in the trial itself.[22] Decision analysis is also useful when a clinical problem requires input from more than one set of study results. For example, the effects of hormone replacement therapy have been analysed in many different studies, each concerned with different outcomes and values.[23] Furthermore, observational studies have shown that women have different baseline risks (for example, thin women are at high risk of fractures). Decision analysis has shown how these factors may be integrated to optimise individual therapy.[24]

Decision analysis is used to work out how to maximise an individual's expected utilities. By obtaining median utilities from a large number of people, the methodology can be used to derive expected utilities at the community level. If the costs of various options are included, this is called a cost utility analysis. However, the use of group median utilities creates some thorny ethical issues where, for example, maximising utility and equity conflict.

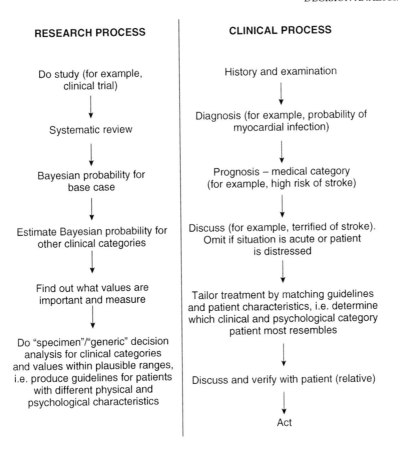

RESEARCH PROCESS	CLINICAL PROCESS

Figure 12.3 Idealised scheme showing (1) how the research process should extend to producing probalistic evidence, specimen values, and (on this basis) generic decision analysis (guidelines); (2) how the clinical process "converges" on a particular guideline. If people had more time then decision analysis could be done more precisely for each patient.

Decision analysis and resource allocation

Decision analysis can help a patient and their physician decide what treatment to give from within the available range. However, it can be extended to help those who commission services decide which treatments should be made available, i.e. to help decisions affecting groups rather than individuals.[20] For example, should insurers, health maintenance organisations, or health authorities fund the availability of tPA (versus SK), or would any marginal money be better spent on another service, say promoting a low salt diet or enhancing an organ transplantation programme. For people like our patients with MI, the expected gains from

149

tPA versus SK vary from SK better and cheaper, tPA better clinically but the gains are small so it is very bad value for money, to tPA so much better that it is a reasonable buy. When something is better in both clinical and economic terms, that alternative is "dominant". For example, colposcopy is not only safer than repeat smear in cases of mildly abnormal cervical cytology, but it is also probably cheaper, thanks to the high proportion who eventually come to colposcopy either way.[25] Decisions may also be dominant in the sense that both the individual and society as a whole loses. For example, screening for prostate cancer stands to add about six months of life to elderly men. However, the treatment (which will often be administered to men who would otherwise die with, but not from, the disease) has many side-effects whose (dis)utilities have been measured. When these are factored into a decision analysis model, a screening programme stands to subtract four months of quality-adjusted life, despite potential gains in longevity. Clearly, a randomised trial to measure the effects of screening on mortality, with slightly greater precision than has been available hitherto, is unlikely to be a cost-effective investment given current therapy for the presymptomatic disease.[26,27] The situation would be quite different if a less morbid form of therapy, such as brachytherapy, were invoked for screen-positive cases. Of course, the more common, interesting, and problematic situation is where an intervention both increases cost and improves health (for example, quality-adjusted life expectancy). In that situation, one calculates the *marginal cost-effectiveness ratio*, which expresses how much needs to be spent to gain each additional quality-adjusted life year (QALY). This was done elegantly with respect to clot-busting drugs by Kellett and Clarke[7] in their article which we cited above. These ratios can be compared one to another in choosing among strategic uses of the health care "pound". Thus, decision analysis provides the (expected) utilities (QALYs) in cost utility analysis. The values now are not individual values but "average" (preferably median) group values. More detail concerning use of group utilities in decision making are given elsewhere.[28–31]

Decision analysis in research design

This chapter has been concerned with the bridge from research findings to decisions. It is worth pointing out, however, that the bridge can also be crossed in the other direction. Intended decisions or envisaged actions can point to design requirements for research. Thus, in addition to modelling the outputs of research, decision analysis is also crucial at the planning stage.

Decision analysis can inform power calculations.[32–34] By making trade-offs explicit, the size of clinical effect that might be useful to patients and clinicians in their decision making can be calculated. For example the trials

150

of small versus large operations for early breast cancer, even when combined,[35] were too small to show the benefits in mortality that women might wish to trade-off against disfigurement and the other complications of more extensive surgery.[36] A decision-analytic model showed that a proposed randomised trial of antenatal tests of fetal well-being was unlikely to produce clear results – realistic gains were most unlikely to be demonstrated by traditional statistical analysis of a trial because plausible gains were so small in absolute numerical terms.[37] On the other hand, Parsonnet and colleagues[38] showed, by means of a study of the relevant epidemiology and decision analysis, that cost-effective gains were plausible from *H. pylori* screening to prevent stomach cancer, and hence that a trial would be a useful investment. Mason and colleagues showed that the decision to screen for abdominal aortic aneurysms would rationally turn on data within the zone of current uncertainty.[39] Indeed, decision analysis at the design stage may include a monetary dimension. For example, Drummond and colleagues[40] conducted an analysis of the Diabetic Retinopathy Study, a major trial funded by the U.S. National Eye Institute. The trial cost $10·5 million, but estimated savings contingent on the knowledge gained amounted to $2816 million, arising in part from enhanced production resulting from a gain of 279 000 vision years.

In addition to sizing clinical studies and justifying their performance, decision analysis, when applied prospectively to a problem, can help inform which of a multitude of trials should be performed (i.e. where additional, relatively "expensive" data would better inform either health policy or decisions for individual patients).

Conclusion: evidence-based care requires a decision analytic framework

Enormous effort is applied to the production of knowledge, but its use is frequently unsystematic and intuitive. Clinical trials and meta-analyses are carried out with minute attention to detail, then the results are applied in a way which is totally informal, idiosyncratic, and opaque. After slavishly crossing every t and dotting every i within research protocols results are simply "taken into account" when decisions are made. If evidence-based care is to be seen through to its logical conclusion, and if both empiric evidence and human values are to be incorporated within the decision making process, then this inconsistency in approach should be tackled.[41,42]

Building better bridges to get from knowledge to action therefore seems the next logical step for the evidence-based movement, and follows rationally from the science of structured reviews and meta-analysis.[18]

151

References

1 Glasziou PP, Irwig LM. An evidence based approach to individualising treatment. *BMJ* 1995;**311**:1356–9.

2 Keeney RL, Raiffa H. *Decisions with multiple objectives.* London: Wiley, 1976.

3 Weinstein M, Fineberg HV. *Clinical decision analysis.* London: Saunders, 1980.

4 French S. *Readings in decision analysis.* London: Chapman and Hall, 1989.

5 Sox HC, Blatt MA, Higgins MC, Marton KI. *Medical decision making.* Boston: Butterworth Heinemann, 1988.

6 ISIS-2 collaborative group. Randomised trial of intravenous streptokinase, oral aspirin, both, or neither among 17 187 cases of suspected myocardial infarction: ISIS-2. *Lancet* 1988;**II**(8607):349–60.

7 Kellett J, Clarke J. Comparison of accelerated tissue plasminogen activator with streptokinase for treatment of suspected myocardial infarction. *Medical Decision Making* 1995;**15**:297–310.

8 Tsevat J, Goldman L, Lamas GA. Functional status versus utilities in survivors of myocardial infarction. *Med Care* 1991;**29**:1153–9.

9 Beck R, Salem DN, Estes NAM, Pauker SG. A computer-based Markov decision analysis of the management of symptomatic bifascicular block: the threshold probability for pacing. *J Am Coll Cardiol* 1987;**9**:920–35.

10 Moser H. Duchenne muscular dystrophy: pathogenic aspects and genetic prevention. *Hum Gen* 1984;**66**:17–40.

11 Lilford RJ, Braunholtz D. The statistical basis of public policy: a paradigm shift is overdue. *BMJ* 1996;**313**:603–7.

12 Goodman SN. Toward evidence-based medical statistics. 2. The Bayes factal. *Ann Intern Med* 1999;**130**:1005–13.

13 Brophy JM, Josph L. Placing trials in context using Bayesian analyses. Gusto, revisited by Reverend Bayes. *JAMA*;**273**:871–5.

14 Donner A. A Bayesian approach to the interpretation of sub-group results in clinical trials. *J Chron Dis* 1982;**34**:429–35.

15 Oxman AD, Guyatt GH. A consumer's guide to sub-group analyses. *Ann Intern Med* 1992;**116**:78–84.

16 Swales J. Science in a health service. *Lancet* 1997;**349**:1319–21.

17 Keeney RL. *Value focused thinking: a path to creative decision making.* Boston: Harvard University Press, 1992.

18 Pettiti DB. *Meta-analysis, decision analysis, and cost-effectiveness analysis methods for quantitative synthesis in medicine.* New York: Oxford University Press, 1994.

19 Thornton J, Lilford RJ, Johnson N. Decision analysis in medicine. *BMJ* 1992;**304**: 1099–103.

20 Thornton J, Lilford RJ. Decision analysis for medical managers. *BMJ* 1995;**310**:791–4.

21 McNeil BJ, Weichselbaum R, Pauker SG. Speech and survival: trade-offs between quality and quantity of life in laryngeal cancer. *New Eng J Med* 1981;**305**:982–7.

22 Sculpher M, Michaels J, McKenna M, Minor J. A cost-utility analysis of laser-assisted angioplasty for peripheral arterial occlusions. *Int J Tech Assess Health Care* 1996;**12**:104–25.

23 Johnson N, Lilford RJ, Mayers D, Johnson GG, Johnson JM. Do healthy, asymptomatic, post-menopausal women want routine cyclical hormone replacement? A utility analysis. *J Obs Gyn* 1994;**14**:35–9.

24 Col NF, Eckman MH, Karas RH *et al.* Patient-specific decisions about hormone replacement therapy in postmenopausal women. *JAMA* 1991;**277**(14):1140–7.

25 Johnson N, Sutton J, Thornton JG, Lilford RJ, Johnson VA, Peel KR. Decision analysis for best management of mildly dyskaryotic smear. *Lancet* 1993;**342**:91–6.

26 Cantor SB, Spann SJ, Volk RJ, Cardenas MP, Warren MM. Prostate cancer screening: a decision analysis. *J Fam Pract* 1995;**41**(1):188–9.

27 Krahn M, Mahoney J, Eckman M, Trachtenberg J, Pauker SG, Detsky AS. Screening for prostatic cancer: a decision-analytic view. *JAMA* 1994;**272**:773–80.

28 Arrow KJ. *Social choice and individual values.* New Haven and London: Yale University Press, 1951.

29 Hudson P, Peel V. Ethical priority setting in the NHS – avoiding playing with numbers. *Br J Health Care Man* 1995;**1**:451–4.

30 Wagstaff A. QALYs and the equity-efficiency trade-off. *J Health Econ* 1991;**10**:21–41.

31 Williams A. *Interpersonal comparisons of welfare*. Discussion paper 151. University of York: Centre for Health Economics, 1996.

32 Thompson M. Decision-analytic determination of study size. *Medical Decision Making* 1981;**1**:165–79.

33 Lilford RJ, Johnson N. The alpha and beta errors in randomised trials. *New Engl J Med* 1990;**322**:780–1.

34 Lilford RJ, Thornton J. Decision logic in medical practice. *J Roy Coll Phys* 1992;**26**:1–20.

35 Early Breast Cancer Trialists' Collaborative Group. Effects of radiotherapy and surgery in early breast cancer: an overview of randomised trials. *New Eng J Med* 1995;**333**:1444–55.

36 Lilford RJ. Clinical trial numbers. *Lancet* 1990;**335**:483–4.

37 De Bono M, Fawdry RDS, Lilford RJ. Size of trials for evaluation of antenatal tests of fetal wellbeing in high-risk pregnancy. *J Perinat Med* 1990;**18**:77–87.

38 Parsonnet J, Harris RA, Hack HM, Owens DK. Modelling cost-effectiveness of *Helicobactor pylori* screening to prevent gastric cancer: a mandate for clinical trials. *Lancet* 1996;**348**:150–4.

39 Mason JM, Wakeman AP, Drummond MF, Crump BJ. Population screening for abdominal aortic aneurysm: do the benefits outweigh the costs? *J Public Health Med* 1993;**15**:2,154–60.

40 Drummond MF, Davies LM, Ferris FL. Assessing the costs and benefits of medical research: the diabetic retinopathy study. *Soc Sci Med* 1992;**34**:973–81.

41 Dowie J. "Evidence based", "cost-effective", and "preference-driven" medicine: decision analysis-based medical decision making is the prerequisite. *J Health Serv Res Policy* 1996; **1**:2,104–13.

42 Dowie J. The research-practice gap and the role of decision analysis in closing it. *Health Care Analysis* 1996;**4**:5–18.

13 Evidence-based policy making

J A MUIR GRAY

Key messages

- Policy making is influenced by resources, values and evidence.
- Evidence-based decision making has led to values becoming much more exposed.
- Increasing pressure on resources and a better educated population means that decision making will be much tougher in the future.
- Policy making will increasingly be evidence-based.

What influences policy?

The term "policy" is defined in the *Shorter Oxford English Dictionary* as "a course of action adopted and pursued by a government, party, ruler, statesman; any course of action adopted as advantageous or expedient". Politics, with the same root, is defined as "relating to the principles, opinions, or sympathies of a person or party."

Yet, despite its political connotations rooted in beliefs and values, "policy" is also used more broadly, for example as "managerial policy" or "clinical policy." With this broader usage, a policy may be defined as "a course of action that an authority states should be followed." Figure 13.1 illustrates the different, overlapping factors that influence policy decisions.

Values and beliefs

Different kinds of values and beliefs influence policy makers. Some relate to prevailing ideological beliefs, which, while sometimes presented as polar opposites, often lie on a continuum. Such different prevailing ideological beliefs would appear to underpin differences in screening policy between the United States and Canada. In the United States, policy making is guided by concern with individuals' rights to make decisions, whereas in Canada, policy making tends to be more influenced by the values of

154

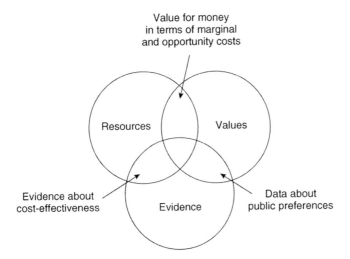

Figure 13.1 Venn diagram showing the three main factors that influence policy making: resources, values, and evidence.

solidarity and community benefit.[1] How these beliefs are applied in policy is illustrated by the countries' respective decisions to perform routine mammographic screening for women younger than 50 years of age.

The Alice in Wonderland of breast cancer screening

The name "Bethesda" is revered in the scientific community because it is the site of the National Institutes of Health (NIH). At its Consensus Conference, NIH panel members used research evidence to conclude that routine mammography was not indicated for women younger than 50. The press, however, ignored the scientific evidence on which the decision was based and attacked both the decision and panel that made it.[2] Congress called for screening for younger women to be introduced. The Director of the NIH National Cancer Institute said that he was "shocked" by the report[3] and asked the Institute's 18-member advisory board to review the evidence. They voted by 17 to 1 to recommend screening for women under 50 years of age.[4]

By contrast, in Canada, there is no routine screening for women younger than 50. There, it is defended on the grounds that research finds no benefit in this age group.

Beneath these differences in approach lies a different understanding about responsibility and choice of health care. In the United States, breast screening is made available to younger women on the grounds that it leaves the decision to individual women who can include it in their insurance coverage or pay for screening themselves, taking advice from their country's most respected clinical research centre. In the final advice from NIH, such focus on individual responsibility overrode the health needs of poorer people and those of the population as a whole.

In Canada and the United Kingdom, however, health is considered as both a community and individual responsibility. Therefore, any benefit enjoyed by a small number of people who may be helped by screening needs to be offset by the impact that such a decision would have on the population as a whole, taking into account both the health and so opportunity costs that introducing breast screening in women younger than 50 would entail.

Evidence- and value-based decision making

One of the main consequences of promoting evidence-based decision making has been to clarify the distinction between values and evidence. Before evidence-based decision making became a powerful paradigm, decisions were made on a combination of opinions and resources. Identifying evidence has led to focus on the two different elements of opinions: propositions supported by evidence and value judgements, now being more clearly exposed. Thus the move to evidence-based decision making has also led to values becoming much more explicit and exposed.

In future, decisions are not simply likely to be about whether or not to fund a new intervention or stop an existing intervention. Health care decision making does not take place on a blank sheet of paper. All health care budgets are fully committed and decisions always take place at the margins. Thus the values likely to be exposed are those concerning change at the margin. The decision whether or not to increase investment in, for example, Down's syndrome screening will inevitably raise issues about where the money is to be found to make such investment. Should it come from within the budget for antenatal services, and, if so, what are the values that should be used to decide on areas for disinvestment?

Alternatively, should it come from some other health care programmes, for example by reducing the amount of money spent on hip replacement, coronary artery bypass grafting, or some other intervention for older people? This would again expose the values that have to be addressed in shifting resources from one group in the population to another.

The analysis of evidence has opened one black box in healthcare decisions; in doing so it has revealed another black box, the black box of values and preferences, and it is this aspect of decision making that will dominate the next phase of evidence-based policy making.

Resources

Resources – both finance and skills – are important for policies to be deliverable and may lead to policies being reviewed.

Evidence about resources

When resources get tight and new options are considered, then evidence may be assembled to appraise the costs and benefits of different policy options. Cost-benefit appraisal was developed primarily by economists, and terms such as cost-benefit analysis, cost-effectiveness analysis, and decision analysis are increasingly used in policy making both by politicians and by managers. New options for encouraging implementation of results from economic evaluations to promote the uptake of research findings are discussed in Chapter 15.

A related technique called "decision analysis" is also increasingly popular (see Chapter 12). In decision analysis, for example, an algorithm has been developed for screening for Down's syndrome, which shows the likely effects of making different decisions. Usually, the algorithm includes value judgements about the beneficial or adverse effects of different options.[5]

In both kinds of techniques, it is customary to use sensitivity analysis, for example to determine what would happen to the analysis and its conclusions if any of the variables changed significantly.

Evidence

Evidence drawn from research and other forms of collected data, such as population-based statistics, increasingly affects policies, although not always in a uniform way.

Policies to protect and promote health

Some policies designed to *protect* people from harm by third parties are a traditional role of the State. Many of these policies, such as those designed to protect individuals from pollution, are usually less strongly opposed and may require a lower level of strength of evidence than health promotion policies. Yet turning them into law can be difficult because of deep-seated opposition to paternalism. Typically, therefore, legislation requires much stronger evidence before it can be introduced, particularly when paternalistic legislation designed to protect one group may harm others.

Seat-belts
This was a crucial issue in the debate before seat-belts were made compulsory in the United Kingdom. Opponents of seat-belt legislation argued not only that it was ethically wrong for the State to force individuals to do anything for their own good (using JS Mill's essay *On Liberty*[6] to support their argument), they also produced evidence that some people were harmed as a result of wearing seat-belts, for example by being unable to get clear of a car in water or on fire. The evidence for the protective effect of

157

seat-belts was strong, but the evidence suggesting that some people would be harmed so that others might live was emotive, and it was not until yet more evidence was produced that the main reason why individuals were unable to escape from crashes was not through wearing seat-belts but by being unconscious that resulted from failing to wear a seat-belt that the argument started to turn.

Children

Different standards are often applied to policy and legislation designed to protect children. The United States has introduced a number of measures to control smoking, ostensibly to benefit children, but these same measures could also be helpful to adults.

Policies about healthcare

Healthcare policies govern the funding and organisation of health services. Traditionally, new healthcare policies have been less frequently based on evidence than policies about health. One reason for this is that health service research is often less generalisable than health research. For example, experiments with health maintenance organisations in the United States are less easy to generalise from than research on new vaccines. There are a growing number of examples, however, where new evidence has led to new policies, particularly in the United Kingdom.

In the UK, the National Screening Committee (www.nsc.nhs.uk) has served this function for the last four years. The Committee began by taking systematic reviews as they were produced by the Medical Research Council and National Health Service Research and Development programme. Table 13.1 shows how each systematic review was used to create policy, sometimes to start a screening programme, sometimes to amend it, and sometimes to call for more research. Such systematic transformation of evidence into practice is possible for the Committee, as it covers a relatively restricted field and is willing to take evidence this seriously.

Another way that the Committee puts evidence into practice is to reach back into the research process, specifying the research questions they would like addressed and the methods they would like used to appraise new technology. Increasingly they are specifying precisely how they would like the results of the research expressed.

Similarly, research workers continue to be involved in the screening policy after the policy decision has been made, able to help the policy makers when some new piece of evidence appears. The change from policy making as a passive recipient of research outputs to the involvement of policy making in specifying and shaping research, allowing in turn research workers to influence policy, has created a powerful new force.

158

Table 13.1 Examples of evidence about health care transformed into policy.

Health Technology Assessment publications	National Screening Committee action
Diagnosis, management and screening of early localised prostate cancer, 1997 (two reports).	On the basis of these reports, the Department of Health issued a letter stating that prostate cancer screening should not be offered until new evidence was available.
Screening for fragile X syndrome, 1997.	The NSC recommended that this should not be introduced.
Neonatal screening for inborn errors of metabolism: cost, yield and outcome 1997 (two reports)	On the basis of these two reports, the NSC's recommendation was that tandem mass spectometry screening should not be introduced as a generic service but that further work should be done to review the evidence about the costs and benefits of screening for specific diseases.
Pre-school vision screening, 1997.	On the basis of this report, the NSC conducted a major review of vision screening and although there was no clear evidence of benefit decided to support the retention of a simplified service with better training of staff.
A critical review of the role of neonatal hearing screening in the detection of congenital hearing impairment, 1997.	The NSC recommended the introduction of universal neonatal hearing screening using auto-acoustic technology to replace the distraction test currently offered by health visitors.
Screening for speech and language delay: a systematic review of the literature, 1998.	On the basis of this report, the NSC recommended that there should not be a national programme of screening for speech and language delay, principally because of the uncertainty about natural history.
Antenatal screening for Down's syndrome, 1998. Ultrasound screening in pregnancy: a systematic review of the clinical effectiveness, cost-effectiveness and women's views, 2000.	The NSC recommended the introduction of a national programme to ensure that all pregnant women were offered a test and follow-up which met explicit quality criteria. This was linked to recommendations about ultrasound screening in pregnancy to minimise variations and quality problems.
Screening for ovarian cancer: a systematic review, 1998.	On the basis of this review, the NSC supported a randomised controlled trial of screening for ovarian cancer which was subsequently funded by the Medical Research Council.
Detection, adherence and control of hypertension for the prevention of stroke: a systematic review, 1998.	A second report on hypertension is expected and the NSC will consider these two reports in 2001.
Screening for cystic fibrosis, 1999.	On the basis of this report, the feasibility of national roll-out of an antenatal screening programme, currently on offer only in Edinburgh and the Lothians, is being explored. Those commissioning health services were recommended not to fund neonatal screening for cystic fibrosis but the publication of a report from the major randomised controlled trial of screening for cystic fibrosis in 2001 led the NSC to review its recommendations.

continued

159

Table 13.1 *(continued)*

Health Technology Assessment publications	National Screening Committee action
A systematic review of the role of human papillomavirus testing within a cervical screening programme, 1999.	On the basis of this report, the NSC recommended a pilot study to assess the practicability of using HPV testing to improve the management of women with equivocal smear results.
Antenatal and neonatal haemoglobinopathy in the UK: review and economic analysis, 1999 (two reports).	A national programme of screening for sickle cell disease and thalassaemia is being introduced on the basis of these reports.
Screening for hypercholesterolaemia versus case finding for familial hypercholesterolaemia: a systematic review and cost-effectiveness analysis, 2000.	On the basis of this report, the NSC has recommended a systematic approach to case finding for hypercholesterolaemia in preference to whole population screening.

Future trends in evidence-based policy making

Predicting policy making is hazardous and perhaps unwise. However, two trends can be discerned in most countries: increasing pressure on resources and a better educated population, more sceptical about the evidence produced by experts.[7] As pressure on resources increases, driven in the health service by rising expectations, population ageing, and new technology, decision makers will have to face tougher decisions. A better educated population will not only have higher expectations of health and other public services but of the decision making process itself, expecting the decisions to be explicit, open, and evidence-based.

The last 50 years has seen a dramatic change in decision making in the UK from an era in which decisions were made by politicians who were primarily lawyers, supported by civil servants who were primarily generalists, particularly in the UK where there was a strong tradition of a Civil Service based on the study of the classics with the scientists within the Civil Service being traditionally accorded lower status. The Second World War changed this, allowing the technocrats to demonstrate what science could do by bringing evidence to decision making; this is brilliantly described in David Halberstam's book *The best and the brightest.*[8] In ministries of health, public health doctors and epidemiologists had brought science and policy making closer together since the latter part of the 19th century but it is only in the last 50 years that evidence-based decision making has become common across all areas of policy making.

In the UK, a conscious decision was taken by policy makers to ensure that 1·5% of the resources made available for patient care should be invested to

160

support research and development. The main reason was to improve the quality and effectiveness of health care by answering questions that health care decision makers – clinicians, managers and patients – were asking and to take explicit steps to ensure that decisions were based on evidence, both through using the performance management system to promote clinical effectiveness and by promoting an evaluative culture designed to make decision makers hungry for best current knowledge which the R&D Programme would provide. This explicit commitment to create an evidence-based health care system emphasised the recognition that policy makers gave to the need for evidence-based decision making.

Epidemiologists can be proud that they were among the first to practise evidence-based decision making, analysing patterns of health and disease to identify the causes of ill health, although the interventions they proposed to tackle these causes were often based on inference and not on hard evidence. For the future it seems certain that the tradition of evidence-based policy making will become increasingly explicit.

Acknowledgements

I am grateful to Emily Gray for contributing the concepts of JS Mill.

References

1 Tanenbaum SJ. "Medical effectiveness" in Canadian and US health policy: the comparative politics of inferential ambiguity. *Health Serv Res* 1996;**31**:5, 517–32.
2 National Cancer Institute. *National Institutes of Health consensus statement: Breast cancer screening for women aged* 40–49. Bethesda, MD: NIH, 1997.
3 Marwick C. NIH consensus panel spurs discontent. *JAMA* 1997;**277**:519–20.
4 Fletcher SW. Whither scientific deliberation in health policy recommendations? Alice in the Wonderland of breast-cancer screening. *N Engl J Med* 1997;**336**:1180–3.
5 Fletcher J, Hicks NR, Kay JDS, Body PA. Using decision analysis to compare policies for antenatal screening for Down's syndrome. *BMJ* 1996;**311**:351–6.
6 Mill JS. *On Liberty*. Fontana Library, 1969.
7 Angell M. *Science on Trial*. New York: WW Norton & Co. Inc., 1996.
8 Halberstam D. *The best and the brightest*. Random House, 1986.

14 Implementing research findings in developing countries

PAUL GARNER, HELEN SMITH, RAJENDRA KALE,
RUMONA DICKSON, TONY DANS,
AND RODRIGO SALINAS

Key messages
- The constraints to implementing research findings into clinical practice in developing countries are varied.
- There is increased use of evidence-based medicine in developing countries.
- Practitioners need access, training and experience with using evidence-based information.

Developing countries have limited resources, so it is particularly important to invest in health care that works. A growing number of relevant systematic reviews can assist policy makers, clinicians, and users in making sensible and informed decisions. Developing countries have led the way in approaches to ensuring standard professional behaviour through guidelines and essential drug programmes. Reliable research summaries can help ensure practice policies are based on good evidence. This chapter examines the constraints to good practice and identifies opportunities that will help translate research into decisions by professionals and users in developing countries in the coming years.

"Wait man bagarapim mi": the colonial legacy

Yakamul, an illiterate villager from Papua New Guinea, was sitting by a fire listening to a health professional from the West tell her to take antimalarial drugs during her pregnancy. She retorted: "I ting merisin bilong ol wait man bai bagarapim mi" (translated: "I think this Western medicine could harm me"). She had not attended a workshop in critical appraisal in Liverpool, Chiang Mai or Manila but appreciated medicine could do her more harm than good. She reminds us to ask fundamental questions about the health care we provide, and of our responsibility to interrogate the evidence using scientific methods. It took us a few years, but eventually we attempted to test her hypothesis.[1]

Making sure we do the right things at the right times is central to translating research into decision making. Practitioners practise in good faith but, if they are wrong, waste resources and can harm people. Nowhere is this more important than in developing countries where many providers struggle to finance accessible health facilities on a budget of less than £7 per person per year.[2] These countries do not have any slack in the system to waste on a single tablet, injection, or activity that is not effective. Equally important is the time and out-of-pocket costs the patients expend on health care. Poor people using ineffective services spend money on services and drugs and remain ill. This means that if we, as health professionals, are responsible collectively for recommending forms of care that are ineffective, then we contribute to deprivation and poverty in the disadvantaged communities of the world.

There are several preconditions for research to be translated into practice; to begin with, the research has to be relevant to decision making. Tropical medicine has a long history of exploitative research that benefited researchers with no direct implications for the participants. For example, a bibliography up to 1977 of research in Papua New Guinea reveals 135 publications describing Melanesian blood groups but only 25 concerned with the treatment of malaria.[3] Descriptive studies are sometimes useful in defining problems, but are of limited value if it is not clear how they might link to interventions. Things are changing, but people in developed countries should not forget their colonial legacy, and some research remains semicolonial.[4]

A second precondition is that research asks sensible questions and is of good quality. We have been surprised by the number of trials we have had to exclude from systematic reviews because the studies address irrelevant questions, are badly designed or of poor quality. In a review of new artemisinin drugs, we excluded 64/105 studies (43%); in the case of impregnated bednets, 47/65 (72%) were excluded; and in the case of headlice treatment, 67/70 (96%) were excluded.[5-7] The substantial waste of resources from poor quality research has been highlighted in the UK, but little discussed in developing countries.[8] This is important to remember when considering the current calls for more investment in research in developing countries, such as the Global Forum for Health Research.[9] This call is timely, but the research has to be high quality and reliable, and to ensure the "capacity building" associated with it is effective.

163

Along with assuming identical standards for the science, we must also avoid pigeon-holing the relevance of the results into the "developing" and the "developed" world. Globalisation has helped us perceive the world as a whole, then consider local differences; and life has changed to make the dichotomy it represents old-fashioned. Now resources for health care in Thailand are more akin to Greece than to Kenya, for example; and where the former Soviet Union fits in to the developing-developed split is not clear. For research, we consider evidence globally, then how particular regional and local factors could influence the interpretation. In this chapter, we use "developing country" as a marker for high levels of poverty and health care need.[10] We appreciate that the label "developing country" is a convenient short cut, but use it cautiously, preferring to specify the countries and regions.

Constraints to good practice

Organisational performance and planning in government services

In theory, well-organised, government-funded health systems in Africa and Asia provide good value for money. The unfortunate truth is that in many countries the systems are inefficient, lack recurrent funds, and employ large numbers of health workers for whom there are no incentives to provide effective care. With systems in such disarray, research-led practice would appear to be irrelevant.

One response to these systemic problems is to identify specific interventions that will save lives, such as oral rehydration salts for children with diarrhoea, or measles vaccines, and set up independent delivery systems for these individual interventions. Superficially this appears to be a good vehicle for delivering evidence-based approaches, but unfortunately the "magic bullets" have sometimes been selected by consensus rather than hard evidence. For example, evidence that growth monitoring prevents malnutrition and infant death is weak, yet every day health staff and mothers spend thousands of hours weighing children.[11] Standard guidelines for antenatal care in many countries still aspire to provide up to 14 visits per pregnancy, although far fewer visits are required in low risk women.[12]

However, even if interventions are evidence-based, a series of vertical programmes may not be the answer. Policy makers, often from international organisations, add more "bullets" to the package, and try to deliver it through a fragmented service. Over time, this process leads to a comprehensive package that the system was not able to deliver in the first place. Then there are attempts to "integrate" delivery,[13] but this may not be effective. The underlying problem of poor organisational performance remains, and the services remain inefficient. Thus evidence-based approaches need to work within systems that are at least functional, or accompany institutional reform that targets organisational performance.

Organisational problems are only a part of the picture facing poorer countries. Political factors are more important. Government per capita allocations to health care may be modest compared to Europe or North America, but the totals are large. As a result, there will always be people with vested interests keen to influence the distribution of funds. Capital investment in new facilities and high technology equipment appeals to politicians and those that vote them in, even when these investments may be the least cost-effective. Corruption and kickbacks create incentives that mitigate against sensible decision making. These problems are universal, but comprehensible evidence of effectiveness could provide some support for those attempting to contradict claims that high technology will cure all.

Unregulated private sector

Outside government, there are further perverse incentives promoting bad practice. Private practitioners sometimes prescribe regimens that are different to, and more expensive than, standard World Health Organization (WHO) guidelines.[14] Knowledge is part of the problem as practitioners in such situations depend on drug representatives for information. Commercial companies have much to gain from promoting drugs, whether they work or not. Because of inadequacies in regulation, these promotional activities often extend beyond ethical limits set by many Western societies. Even worse, at times they may come disguised as a form of continuing medical education. The situation is aggravated by lack of effective policy regarding approval of drugs for marketing. In Pakistan, for example, the lack of any effective legislation means that the authorities register approximately five new pharmaceutical products every day.[15]

Doctors

Ultimately the medical profession is the main constraint to change. In some countries of Asia and Latin America, self-referral and ownership of equipment or hospital facilities is allowed or even condoned by medical societies and training institutions. This creates a conflict of interest, which may explain the irrational overuse of many diagnostic tests. Furthermore, clinicians and public health physicians base their medical knowledge on foreign (mainly European and US) literature and the opinions of foreign visitors, usually supported by drug companies, who are promoting a new product. However, clinicians believe scientific understanding is

165

essential for designing rational treatment; they are respected if they know about the pathology of disease. Medical freedom is valued, and where possible we should avoid strategies to implement research into practice that are perceived as a threat to this.

Opportunities

In the quest for translating research into practice, it is common for researchers, funding organisations and policy makers in Africa, Asia and Latin America to expect a single study within a particular country to directly translate into change and action nationally or locally. This is an unreasonable expectation, and scientifically questionable. To begin with, it is rare that the results of a study are so dramatic that they result in a policy change overnight. One piece of research contributes to a global pool of knowledge, and the study needs to be interpreted in the context of the rest of the available evidence. For research on interventions using randomised controlled trials, then the trial needs to be set in the context of other similar studies to seek consistency of effects, or differences between studies, which might reflect the play of chance, bias or true differences in effects. Overall, then, there is an opportunity to use research synthesis to promote translation of research from the global pool into local contexts. The science around appraising applicability is rapidly developing, and checklists are available to help think through this process.[16]

Large trials and research synthesis in medicine has helped make certainty and uncertainty explicit. The logic for up-to-date global summaries of research evidence is appealing. In our experience, it is attractive to policy makers and clinicians in many countries. So the current climate is ripe. Indeed, national policy makers want to see this happen. In a recent consultation with health policy makers in the West African Region, we found that policy makers wanted research to be relevant to their needs, and to have some say in how research priorities were set in their country. Some Africans with PhDs and research experience have moved to senior policy positions, and this is improving the use of research, as well as the drive to make researchers more accountable.

The wider awareness of evidence-based approaches makes poorly informed decisions increasingly untenable. The previous Director General of the World Health Organization made the mistake of declaring that directly observed therapy for tuberculosis was the greatest advance since penicillin. We challenged WHO repeatedly for the evidence, as it was clear the WHO rhetoric for direct observation was being forced on some countries and damaging existing TB control programmes.[17] The underlying problem was that the intervention was complex, and, in the process of making a global programme, WHO had oversimplified the inputs.[18] The challenge was

166

constructive, as WHO then clarified what they meant by WHO–DOT, which now can include self-treatment by patients at home.

Established and new initiatives

Trainers, policy makers, and clinicians have already done a lot to engender a science-led culture in developing countries. The Rockefeller Foundation has supported training of clinicians in critical appraisal for over 15 years, producing clinicians committed to science-based practice in their countries.[19] Local initiatives raising awareness around evidence-based approaches are springing up in a variety of settings. In Chiang Mai, Manila, and Singapore, evidence-based courses for clinicians have been established. In Nigeria, clinicians in Calabar have set up an evidence-based office, helping people conduct systematic reviews, and promoting their use through clinical services and community organisations, such as the Sickle Cell Club (Meremikwu M, personal communication).

Some national governments are now also taking positive action to introduce research-led practice. The Ministry of Health in Chile has set up an evidence-based health office with support from the European Union, and this has recently expanded to become a national health technology assessment programme. In Thailand, the Ministry of Health and the National Health Systems Research Institute are setting up an evidence-based practice office to guide their national hospital accreditation programme (Supachutikul A, personal communication). In South Africa, the Medical Research Council has committed support for the production of systematic reviews and evidence-based practice (Volmink J, personal communication). In the Philippines, the Department of Health has contributed generously to funding for major projects on evidence-based guideline development, particularly to direct its cardiovascular disease prevention programme.[20]

Practice policies are widely used in Africa and parts of the Pacific, and guidelines have been in use in Papua New Guinea since 1966.[21] Guidelines for acute respiratory illness in children, for example, had an evidence base established years ago.[22] More recently, the methodological tools available for improving validity of these guidelines has increased dramatically. In the Philippines, issues for guideline development were identified, and an approach was proposed that may be used by other developing countries.[23] Furthermore, the WHO Essential Drugs Programme has taken a strong international lead in advocating rational prescribing. Together with the International Network for the Rational Use of Drugs, they have disseminated research about effectiveness. In addition, they have encouraged management interventions that promote good prescribing practice.[24]

Donors and UN organisations concerned with health have clearly influenced the content and direction of health services in developing countries. There are clear indications these groups are now making themselves explicitly evidence-based. The Department for International Development (UK) state in their Health and Population Strategy Paper that "DfID helps make the necessary knowledge available and accessible by ... reviewing evidence from existing sources in a systematic manner, to produce more robust interpretations and guidance on good practice". The Tropical Diseases Research Programme of the World Health Organization has provided the impetus for important reviews in malaria,[5,25] and has committed to an individual patient data analysis of trials testing artesunate combined with existing antimalarial drugs for treating malaria. The World Health Organization are now commissioning reviews, such as the review of low osmolarity oral rehydration solution for diarrhoea,[26] and the Global Filariasis Eradication Programme has commissioned a suite of reviews about interventions for filariasis.

Evidence of effectiveness is capturing the attention of some health care user organisations. The Network for the Rational Use of Medication in Pakistan is launching a consumer journal to help develop community pressure against poor pharmaceutical and prescribing practice. In India, inclusion of medical services under the Consumer Protection Act has increased the accountability of doctors and made patients, especially in the urban areas, more aware of their rights as consumers.

Future directions

Access

We began this chapter by pointing out that research summaries are often a necessary prerequisite for an individual attempting to make sense of available evidence that is buried under a mass of conflicting opinion. The next prerequisite is to ensure that people in developing countries have access to up-to-date information (see Box 14.1). It is important to disseminate to a variety of audiences, including other professionals, the intelligent lay reader, and journalists, but efforts to do so in developing countries require further development and evaluation.

Improving access to the world wide web is central to increasing the "information flow" of reliable medical evidence both to and within resource poor countries.[27] Investment in technology infrastructure through international donors is helping to improve access, but publishers of medical information also have a significant role to play. Given the high cost of internet use, people need free access to electronic journals and published research. The appearance of barrier free access information servers, such as

---

Box 14.1   Strategy to induce change in obstetric care in hospitals

The purpose of the Better Births Initiative is to improve maternity care by:
1 Identifying specific changes that are achievable, and could dramatically improve women's experiences during labour.
Specific changes identified include:
- Encouraging a partner, friend relative or lay carer to support women during labour
- Stopping routine procedures that are of no proven benefit, particularly if they are embarrassing or uncomfortable (for example, shaving, supine position for birth)
- Avoiding making interventions routine where there is no evidence of benefit. This includes: routine enemas, routine restriction to bed, routine intravenous fluids, and routine episiotomy.
2 Developing and testing innovative methods to bring about these changes.
3 Developing an agreed strategy (the Better Births Initiative) which is simple, accessible and applicable to low-income countries.
4 Implementing the strategy in local spheres of influence.
5 Encouraging others to adopt the package.

BioMed Central,[28] has a great potential to contribute to increasing the supply of information to low-income settings. An added advantage of downloading from free electronic sources is that information can then be distributed more widely through national and regional resource centres.[29] In addition, the World Health Organization Reproductive Health Library, which contains a selected number of Cochrane reviews, is published annually and distributed free to health workers in developing countries.[30] However, there is a long way to go in ensuring adequate dissemination.

Training and projects

We know from good systematic reviews that simple access to information is unlikely in itself to change practice, and that change needs some kind of organisational process to help make it happen. Haynes and Haines in Chapter 10 point out some of the barriers to change, and Hunt discussed barriers in relation to nurses, although this could apply to us all. Practitioners do not use research because they do not know about the findings; they don't understand them; they don't believe them; they don't know how to use them; or they are not allowed to use them.[31]

There is certainly a need to communicate to practitioners and policy makers the principles of critical appraisal, and the need for considering

169

reliable evidence in their decisions. This might initially be through special workshops, but in time needs mainstreaming into the training of health professionals. There is an increasing awareness that using research in practice is not a mechanical, simple process of implementing review findings. There is often considerable uncertainty, and other factors to take into account. Even asking students to decide on best practice using systematic reviews yielded a wide range of options, and people need to develop skills and experience in using reliable research in policies and practice.[32]

We should be optimistic. Many mechanisms to implement good practices are already available and well-rehearsed in developing countries. In some, guidelines and standard treatment manuals are better developed than in the West. These guidelines are likely to become more evidence-based over time, as there is little point in effective implementation of ineffective interventions.

These mechanisms must be integrated into service policy and management as a whole, using a layered approach. For example, in June 1995, a large trial showed that magnesium sulphate was the most effective treatment of eclampsia. At that time, one-third of the world's obstetric practice was using other, less effective therapies.[33] The international layer begins with the World Health Organization, ensuring they include the drug on their essential drugs list. Nationally, ministries should include the drug in their purchasing arrangements, and ensure that their curricula and clinical guidelines are consistent with the best treatment. At a local level, midwives and doctors need to be aware of its value. Quality assurance programmes and less formal clinical monitoring should include eclampsia treatment in their audit cycles.

Even when key facilitators are in place, at the international and national level, it is at the local level where multiple barriers can prevent the use of evidence in practice. At the point of delivery, established practice patterns must be challenged, and new ones reinforced. Management theory suggests a process of "unfreezing, changing behaviour, and re-freezing" is paramount to successful organisational change.[34] The principle of "unfreezing", combined with a sound vision to help direct change is a useful strategy that can be applied to clinical practice.[35] We have made good progress in evidence-based care during childbirth using this innovative approach. The "Better Births Initiative" is a high profile package that uses interactive materials (including workbooks, posters, video presentations, and self-audit) and is being tested in educational workshops with midwives in South Africa (see Box 14.1).[36]

Aside from addressing the need for information dissemination, policy makers must also address the hindrances to wider acceptance of evidence and evidence-based guidelines. In particular, policies on ethical drug promotion should be drafted and strictly implemented, as well as policies governing "continuing medical education" and ownership of medical equipment.

Policy

In 1993, the World Bank constructed the "essential package" of effective healthcare interventions. They made many assumptions in the estimates of effectiveness, and in the main did not use systematic reviews as there were very few available.[37] However, the global attention on research synthesis means we expect more rigorous attention to research in policy formulation. For example, their antihelminth policy for school children was judged by the the World Bank in 1993 to be "extremely cost-effective", but a recent systematic review questioned whether the optimism for benefit was fully grounded in evidence.[38] There are likely to be increasing opportunities for more rigorous analyses, such as the analysis by Mills and colleagues, which drew extensively on systematic reviews.[39]

In many countries, donors are also promoting health sector reform, consisting of substantial institutional change in government health policies. Although reforms are different in each country[40] the fact that there is change in progress provides the opportunity for introducing evidence-based approaches alongside the institutional and organisational changes.

Given the current momentum, how can we further promote the use of research findings in policy? Whilst intensive communication with policy makers and professionals is important, alongside demonstration projects such as the Better Births Initiative, we should not forget the public. It is the public – irrespective of income or location – who make the ultimate decision whether to avail themselves of our care or advice.

Paradoxically, people living in developing countries are sometimes the most critical. Yakamul was from a tribe that was poor: life was full of risks, time was always short. The villagers were not afraid to be selective about the components they valued from both the traditional and Western health systems.[41] As health professionals, we should remember that the public also needs information about effectiveness. In communicating this, we should be honest, humble, and explicit when there is uncertainty in the available evidence.

Footnote

This chapter represents the work of the Effective Health Care Alliance Programme, a network of individuals with common objectives around research synthesis and translating research into practice in middle and low-income countries. The Alliance helps people prepare and maintain systematic reviews in relevant health problems, as part of the Cochrane Collaboration; it promotes the dissemination of the information; and it helps stimulate change, with local initiatives, research and trials to influence provider behaviour. A key feature of the programme is collaborative research and implementation between countries, and the Alliance includes people in Chile, China, Ghana, Nigeria, Pakistan, South Africa and Thailand. It is co-ordinated from Liverpool, UK, and supported by the Department for International Development (UK).

The first edition of this chapter was drafted and completed by Paul Garner and Rajendra Kale, with help from Rumona Dickson, Tony Dans and Rodrigo Salinas. The second edition was updated by Paul Garner and Helen Smith.

References

1 Garner P, Gülmezoglu AM. Prevention versus treatment for malaria in pregnant women (Cochrane Review). In: *The Cochrane Library*, Issue 1, 2001. Oxford: Update Software.
2 National Audit Office. *Overseas development administration: health and population overseas aid*. Report by the Comptroller and Auditor General. CH 782 Session 1994–5. London: HMSO, 1995.
3 Homabrook RW, Skeldon GHE. *A bibliography of medicine and human biology of Papua New Guinea*. Monograph Series No. 5. Goroka: Papua New Guinea Institute of Medical Research, 1977.
4 Costello A, Zumla A. Moving to research partnerships in developing countries. *BMJ* 2000; **321**:827–9.
5 McIntosh HM, Olliaro P. Artemisinin derivatives for treating uncomplicated malaria (Cochrane Review). In: *The Cochrane Library*, Issue 4, 2000. Oxford: Update Software.
6 Lengeler C. Insecticide-treated bednets and curtains for preventing malaria (Cochrane Review). In: *The Cochrane Library*, Issue 4, 2000. Oxford: Update Software.
7 Dodd CS. Interventions for treating headlice (Cochrane Review). In: *The Cochrane Library*, Issue 4, 2000. Oxford: Update Software.
8 Altman DG. The scandal of poor medical research. *BMJ* 1993;**308**:283–4.
9 Global Forum for Health Research. *The 10/90 Report on Health Research 2000*. Geneva: World Health Organization, 2000.
10 Garner P, Kiani A, Salinas R, Zaat J. Effective health care [letter]. *Lancet* 1996;**347**:113.
11 Panpanich R, Garner P. Growth monitoring in children (Cochrane Review). In: *The Cochrane Library*, Issue 3, 2000. Oxford: Update Software.
12 Villar J, Khan-Neelofur D. Patterns of routine antenatal care for low-risk pregnancy (Cochrane Review). In: *The Cochrane Library*, Issue 3, 2000. Oxford: Update Software.
13 Briggs J. Strategies for integrating primary health services (Cochrane Protocol). In: *The Cochrane Library*, Issue 1, 2001: Oxford: Update Software.
14 Uplekar MW, Rangan S. Private doctors and tuberculosis control in India. *Tuber Lung Dis* 1993;**74**:332–7.
15 Bhutta TI, Mirza Z, Kjani A. 5.5 new drugs per day! *The Newsletter*. Islamabad: the Association for Rational Use of Medication in Pakistan, 1995;**4**:3.
16 Dans AL, Dans LF. Introduction to EBM in developing countries. www.library.utoronto.ca/medicine/ebm/syllabi/devl/intro.htm
17 Volmink J, Garner P. Directly observed therapy. *Lancet* 1997;**349**:1399–400.
18 Volmink J, Matchaba P, Garner P. Directly observed therapy and treatment adherence. *Lancet* 2000;**355**:1345–50. 1701 [systematic review].
19 Halstead SB, Tugwell P, Bennett K. The international clinical epidemiology network (INCLEN): a progress report. *J Clin Epidemiol* 1991;**44**:579–89.
20 Multisectoral task force on the detection and management of hypertension. Philippine guidelines on the detection and management of hypertension. *Phil J Intern Med* **35**(2): 67–85.
21 Biddulph J. Standard regimens – a personal account of the Papua New Guinea experience. *Trop Doct* 1989;**19**:126–30.

22 Shann F, Hart K, Thornas D. Acute lower respiratory tract infections in children: possible criteria for selection of patients for antibiotic therapy and hospital admission. *Bull WHO* 1984;**62**:749–53.

23 Tumanan BA, Dans AL *et al.* Hypercholesterolemia guidelines development cycle. *Phil Cardiol* 1996;**24**(4):147–50.

24 Interim Report of the Biennium 1996–1997. *Action programme on essential drugs*. Geneva: World Health Organization, 1997.

25 Olliaro P, Nevill C, Ringwald P, Mussano P, Gamer P, Brasseur P. Systematic review of amodiaquine treatment in uncomplicated malaria. *Lancet* 1996;**348**:1196–201.

26 Kim Y, Hahn S, Garner P. Reduced osmolarity oral rehydration solution for treating dehydration caused by acute diarrhoea in children (Protocol for a Cochrane Review). In: *The Cochrane Library*, Issue 2, 2001. Oxford: Update Software.

27 Godlee F, Horton R, Smith R. Global information flow. *BMJ* 2000;**321**:776–7.

28 www.biomedcentral.com

29 Patrikios H. Internet access is not yet universal [response]. *BMJ* 2001;**322**:172.

30 Gulmezoglu M, Villar J, Carroli G *et al.* WHO is producing a reproductive health library for developing countries [letter]. *BMJ* 1997;**314**:1695.

31 Hunt JM. Barriers to research utilization. *J Adv Nurs* 1996;**23**:423–5.

32 Dickson R, Abdullahi W, Flores W *et al.* Putting evidence into practice. *World Health Forum* 1998;**19**:311–14.

33 Eclampsia Trial Collaborative Group. Which anticonvulsant for women with eclampsia? Evidence from the Collaborative Eclampsia Trial. *Lancet* 1995;**345**:1455–63

34 Eisenburg JM. *Doctors' decisions and the cost of medical care*. Michigan: Health Administration Press, 1986.

35 Kotter JK. Leading change: why transformation efforts fail. *Harv Bus Rev* 1985; March–April.

36 http://www.liv.ac.uk/lstm/bbimainpage.html

37 World Bank. *World Development Report 1993: investing in health*. Washington: Oxford University Press, 1993.

38 Dickson R, Awasthi S, Williamson P, Demellweek C, Garner P. Effects of treating children for intestinal helminths on growth and cognitive performance: a systematic review of randomised trials. *BMJ* 2000;**320**:1697–701 [systematic review].

39 Goodman CA, Coleman PG, Mills A. Cost-effectiveness of malaria control in sub-Saharan Africa. *Lancet* 1999; **354**:378–85.

40 Martinez J, Sandiford P, Gamer P. International transfers of NHS reforms [letter]. *Lancet* 1994;**344**:956.

41 Welsch RL. *The experience of illness among the Ningerum of Papua New Guinea* [PhD dissertation]. Washington: University of Washington, 1982. Available through University Microfilms International, Michigan number 3592.

15 Opportunity costs on trial: new options for encouraging implementation of results from economic evaluations

NEIL CRAIG AND MATTHEW SUTTON

Key messages

A description of the current approach to encouraging implementation

- Prioritising healthcare interventions on the basis of cost and benefit considerations involves a number of important assumptions (see Box 15.1).
- Most economic evaluations adopt a societal perspective and indicate the optimal long-term solution where these assumptions hold.
- Real-life incentives and budget allocation mechanisms do not reflect these assumptions but where possible should be manipulated to do so in the long-term.
- In the short-term, the quality of the evidence in economic evaluations should be improved by standardising methods of analysis and reporting.

New options for encouraging implementation in the short-term

- Decision making takes place within real-life situations in which the resources available, the extent to which resources are fully used, the divisibility and the transferability of resources within and between budgets, and the objectives of decision makers differ from place to place and over time.
- In addition, the relationship between costs, effectiveness and volume may not be linear.
- For these reasons, opportunity costs are context-specific.
- Cost-constrained evaluation designs should be adopted to ensure that economic evaluations consider the opportunity costs actually faced by decision makers.
- Some evaluations may need to take place in the context of behavioural analyses of decision making, both to reflect how decision makers react to policy changes and budget constraints in the design of evaluations, and to understand whether and how decision makers use economic information in practice.

Introduction

There are various barriers to the implementation of research findings on the effectiveness of healthcare interventions.[1] Economic evaluation, which relates the costs to the benefits of different interventions, faces similar problems but also appears to face a number of additional challenges. Considerable debate continues within health economics on the fundamentals of analysis.[2–5] Notwithstanding these differences, many have argued for the importance of "standards" in published economic evaluations and progress has recently been made.[6–8] More and better information is available and accessible to a growing number of decision makers and advisors.[8] Yet the evidence suggests that the influence of economics on decision making remains limited, despite the emphasis currently placed on evidence-based medicine and economic information in the NHS.[9–12] Even where there are high quality data and belief in the broad principles upon which health economics is based, there seem to be difficulties in ensuring implementation of the results of economic evaluations over and above those faced by effectiveness studies.[8]

This chapter explores why this may be so and suggests ways in which the issue might be tackled. It highlights the assumptions about priority setting decision making processes that are often implicit in the methods of economic evaluation and discusses the divergence of these assumptions from the context for which the results are intended. It is argued that although the assumptions are valid from a long-term societal perspective, they often cannot be generalised to the short term. As a result, economic evaluation could remain rather peripheral to healthcare decision making unless novel study designs and methods for analysing secondary data are developed which reflect more accurately the contexts in which decisions are made.

The basics of economic evaluation

The scarcity of healthcare resources means that choices have to be made between alternative healthcare interventions. Economic evaluation provides information to enable these choices to be made on the basis of the expected costs and benefits of the alternative treatments which might be made available. The potential benefit from the 'next-best alternative' is the opportunity cost of a particular service. Opportunity cost is often explained in the context of a fixed budget for a healthcare service. Within a fixed budget regime, the decision to implement one option implies that an alternative option cannot also be implemented. Thus, each chosen option has a cost since the benefits of the alternative(s) are not chosen. Opportunity costs therefore provide the rationale for examining the costs

175

as well as the outcomes of interventions.[13] Economic evaluation is not concerned with costs *per se*. "[M]easuring 'costs' ... is only an intermediate step to a comparison of benefits and is of no significance in itself" (Dowie,[14] p.88).

There are a wide range of publications explaining the principles[15,16] and describing the practice[17,18] of economic evaluation. In this chapter it is not intended to rehearse these issues or the rationale for economic evaluation,[13,19] but to consider specifically the important features of economic evaluation which may influence implementation.

It has been shown that following an algorithm based on cost-effectiveness leads to an optimal allocation of resources under a number of conditions[20] (Box 15.1). While economic evaluation can be applied from a variety of perspectives, including patients, providers, health authorities and health boards, government or society as a whole, the societal perspective is advocated as the ideal by most economists,[7,21] with maximisation of the welfare of society as a whole as the objective underlying most economic evaluations.

If we adopt a societal perspective, it is necessary to have information on all potential uses of the resources under study.[4] Since this is not feasible, market prices are proposed as measures of opportunity cost on the assumption that in a perfectly competitive market they represent the value of those resources in their "next-best use". Where healthcare costs differ from those which would be generated by a perfectly competitive market, it is recommended that suitable adjustments be made.[7]

Box 15.1   The basic assumptions of cost-effectiveness[a]

- The decision maker faces a range of options from which to choose.
- There is a fixed budget.
- The decision maker has a well-defined objective which s/he seeks to maximise.
- Any combination of the options is feasible as long as the total costs do not exceed the budget.
- The costs and benefits of each option are independent of which combination is chosen.
- The options are not repeatable.
- All options are fully divisible, i.e. any proportion of any option can be selected.
- All options exhibit constant returns to scale, i.e. costs and benefits rise proportionately with the level of implementation.

[a]Adapted from Weinstein,[83] Box 5.1.

We shall return to discuss the issue of cost data in some detail later but note here that one of the "fundamentals of analysis" upon which economists disagree is the *definition* of "benefit", as distinct from the *measurement* of benefits. Much of economic theory assumes that benefit, or social welfare, should be defined in terms of the utility, or satisfaction, that individuals derive from the consumption of goods and services such as health care. In this so-called "welfarist" approach, social welfare is given by the sum of the utility enjoyed by each individual in society.[22] The source of utility itself generates debate amongst economists, some arguing that utility is derived solely from the impact of health care on states of health, others arguing that the *process* of being screened or treated is itself a source of utility.[23] For example, information derived from screening tests which may reveal no illness or which may reveal illness without influencing patient management is often cited as an example of process utility.

Others have argued for a less individualistic, or extra-welfarist, concept of benefit in which decision makers can pursue health and healthcare objectives which they deem to be in the common good, such as equity, legal restrictions on consumption of drugs or alcohol, or state provision of immunisation, but which may conflict with individual judgements of value.[24] We do not intend to explore this debate in detail but the important points for the current discussion are threefold. Firstly, the benefits measured and the techniques used to do so should be appropriate to the position taken. Secondly, the "correct" position *is* a matter of debate. Economic evaluations, which are more commonly taken from an extra-welfarist perspective,[25] *are* adopting a particular normative position, with which the decision maker using the results of the analyses might not agree. Thirdly, what economics has to offer is not the correct position in this debate, but a systematic way of analysing the costs and benefits of different policy or treatment choices, *whatever* position is taken. Recognition of these issues is necessary both to understand the ethical implications of the results of economic evaluations, and to help understand why the results generated from one perspective may not be taken on board by decision makers adopting a different perspective.

Whatever the definition of benefit adopted, economic evaluations usually compare programmes on the basis of the ratio of costs to benefits. As Birch and Gafni[3] highlight, this requires full divisibility of programmes and constant returns to scale. In other words, any fraction of each intervention can be adopted and the total costs (benefits) of each programme are simply the product of the costs (benefits) per patient and the number of patients treated. On the cost side, it is popular to assume a long-run societal perspective in which all programmes are divisible and marginal costs equal average costs.[7,26] However, on the benefits side, this would imply that the incremental effectiveness of the programme does not change as a larger number of individuals are treated, which is unlikely if patients are selectively

177

prioritised in terms of likely capacity to benefit from services. In this case, programmes should be compared on the basis of the ratio of additional costs to additional benefits (the Incremental Cost-Effectiveness Ratio).[27] However, often it is difficult to compare all feasible options because different comparators are being used for different interventions.[28] In this case, a linear programming approach could be adopted which allows for divisible, partially divisible and indivisible programmes.[29]

However, while we agree that such an exercise may generate the optimal solution in a "first-best" world, there are a number of reasons why it is unlikely to do so in practice and why the results of studies based on this approach may not be adopted in practice. In the next section we discuss why economic information may be rejected before going on to discuss some of the conceptual limitations of the approach and offering an alternative approach later in the chapter.

The current approach to implementing evidence

The Evidence-based Medicine (EBM) Ideal

Attempts to promote the use of economic evaluation in priority setting decisions form an important part of the EBM movement. Improving the standards, accessibility and understanding of research evidence has been the approach adopted. The process by which decisions are made is implicitly assumed to be a model of "consumer" choice. The consumer is the person or organisation responsible for prioritising or choosing between health services. The role of health economics is to provide information on the costs and benefits of competing uses of healthcare resources. The rational consumer wants and will make use of the best information available to optimise their decisions. Based on this model, efforts to promote the use of economic evaluation have concentrated on making more and better information available to increasing numbers of healthcare decision makers.

EBM in practice

Evidence suggests that in practice, decision making processes bear little resemblance to the model of choice implicit in EBM for a number of reasons.[30] Firstly, the process of decision making involves a range of "consumers" in the form of organisations operating at a number of levels. The government defines and influences broad priorities through, *inter alia*, policy statements[31] and executive letters[31,32] to trust and health authority chief executives and GPs, against which performance is measured through a range of accountability review processes. Health authorities have

178

responsibility for establishing local population priorities. Hospitals shape priorities through capital plans and by developing new services. Healthcare professionals establish *de facto* priorities through their treatment and referral decisions.

Secondly, each of these "consumers" may not share a common objective. Maximising health outcomes for the population at large competes with a range of other objectives for both healthcare professionals[33] and the public[34]. A wider variety of information sources are used in making decisions to meet these objectives than the effectiveness and cost-effectiveness research promoted under the auspices of EBM.

Thirdly, even the meaning of shared objectives is contested. For example, studies have suggested that the value to the public of the same benefits, measured in terms of life years saved adjusted for quality of life, differ according to whether the benefits derive from life years saved or improvements in quality of life. It also depends upon whether the service is for chronic or life threatening conditions. Interventions which prolong life appear to be valued more highly.[35,36] In the Oregon experiment, for example, the prioritisation of interventions on the basis of a crude cost utility ratio gave rise to what were considered to be "counter intuitive" priorities in which some interventions for non-acute non-life-threatening conditions were estimated to be more cost-effective than treatments for acute life threatening conditions. The lists were unacceptable and were rejigged. Although the criteria on which this was done were not made explicit, they appeared to reflect the higher priority decision makers felt should be attached to life threatening conditions, irrespective of the cost-effectiveness of the treatments available to treat them.[37,38]

Fourthly, all the groups identified above are not equally powerful in effecting the choices they wish to make. Arguably, the most powerful groups are the Department of Health and healthcare professionals, the former through their influence over health care priorities via the policy and accountability review processes, the latter through their considerable autonomy in deciding how much of what treatment they offer to patients. Ferlie *et al.* "identify tacit expert knowledge as a key power resource in shaping the way research evidence influences clinical practice."[39] The internal market was to change this situation by vesting purchasing power in health authorities and boards who were given responsibility for purchasing services on the public's behalf. In practice, however, health authorities had a more arm's length influence over priorities, more akin to employers who sub-contract to firms who produce services for them, giving only broad indications of the proportion of the budget to be spent on different services. The influence of the health authority as purchaser was undermined further by both the reliance on the sub-contractor for information regarding the cost and quality of the services produced, and by the vested interests of the sub-contractor in the pattern of services delivered. There are a number of such principal-agent relationships involved in the "choice" process determining health care priorities.[40] Imperfections in these arrangements limit the ability of decision makers to ensure their proposals are implemented.

Alternative models of decision making

The net effect of these varied influences on decision making is that the relationship between the evidence base and its diffusion is weak.[39,41] Alternative behavioural frameworks have been developed for explaining why clinician and organisational decision making departs from the rationalist ideal of the EBM movement. Whynes, for example, considers how the notions of benefits and opportunity cost are incorporated into clinicians' decision making behaviour.[42] He models treatment choice as a utility function in which the clinician's utility is a function of benefits, perceived costs, a "coefficient of diagnostic confidence" dependent on the individual clinician's skills and the individual patient's condition, and the personal interests of clinicians in particular treatment choices. Perceived costs are given by:

- The subjective probabilities of each possible outcome
- The expected cost of each outcome
- The physician's view of the importance of the cost of treatment relative to the benefits.

Information on cost-effectiveness influences the subjective probabilities in this model of the treatment decision but it does not necessarily influence the "coefficient of diagnostic confidence", the importance attached to the opportunity cost of the resources involved, the utility derived by the clinician from different outcomes, nor the incentives faced by the clinician to pursue a particular treatment choice. Whynes concludes that "the acquisition of medical evidence can offer only limited scope for harmonising clinical judgements over the desirability of intervention in specific situations."

Escarce considers the diffusion of information and how individual decisions may be influenced by group behaviour.[43] He models the adoption of new treatment technologies and hypothesises that factors which increase the revenue, reduce the costs, or reduce the perceived uncertainty associated with a new technology will increase the speed at which it is adopted. The latter factor is crucial since it is a function of both the economic evidence available, and the attitude to risk of potential adopters. Escarce's empirical results show that clinicians form a heterogeneous group of more or less risk-averse potential adopters whose behaviour is influenced by the availability of information, and by the adoption of new technology

180

by "product champions". Mimicry of "product-champions" may be more efficient than reassessment of the costs and benefits of a particular treatment from the available information.[44] This may suggest that different people respond to different types of information regarding the potential costs and benefits of alternative treatments, some responding to the formal evidence of controlled trials and systematic reviews, others to experiential evidence based on personal or colleagues' use of particular technologies.[30,39]

The current situation

Whether for these or for other reasons, the uptake of the results of economic evaluations by decision makers in the NHS is developing slowly.[9–12] The problems faced in trying to inform priority setting decisions with the results of economic evaluation were graphically illustrated by the Oregon experiment referred to earlier, in which around 600 so-called treatment-condition pairs (TCPs) were ranked according to the ratio of cost to benefit. Costs were based on treatment charges.[37] Benefits were measured in terms of the difference in utility, or quality of life, with and without treatment. Utilities were assessed by telephone surveys of the public using rating scales known to underestimate the utility associated with relatively minor adverse health states. Single cost utility ratios were estimated for broad TCPs including heterogeneous mixes of procedures and patients. Both cost and outcome data in the original list were therefore weak and the list was rejected.

It is unclear, however, whether it was the technical weaknesses or the ethical implications of the rankings which led to their rejection. It is possible that it was both. Clearly, the costs used were not true reflections of opportunity cost. However, as suggested above, the nature of the changes made to subsequent lists suggest that the unacceptability of the rankings per se contributed substantially to the rejection of the original list. In short, both data quality in, and the implications of, economic evaluations are likely to influence their uptake by decision makers.

Drummond et al.[9] address the former issue, suggesting that evidence from economic evaluations may be better incorporated into practice by improving the standard of the information contained in published studies and by changing incentives so that providers are encouraged to adopt a more societal perspective. Contracting and commissioning, for example, were introduced to create a mechanism whereby public health authorities could allocate resources to providers who became more responsive to patients' needs and demands. The *raison d'être* of the internal market was to create the competitive pressures on providers to respond to the choices of agents without a vested interest in current, or indeed in any particular, patterns of resource use. A more effective alternative to changing incentives might be direct measures such as constraining the options available to decision makers by including cost-effectiveness criteria in the licensing of new pharmaceutical products.[45]

However, changing institutions and incentive structures is a complex task. Evidence from the USA suggests that the question is not whether providers respond to financial pressures and incentives, but of whether economic incentives can be designed which encourage clinically and economically appropriate behaviour, avoiding for example cost shifting, cream skimming and premature discharge.[46] In the UK, contracting has not had the radical impact envisaged by its founders,[47,48] and conflicts between cost and quality are not easily resolved.[49] A number of weak and in some cases perverse incentives have been identified in the regulatory regime governing the market[50] which have undermined both the flexibility of resources within the health service and, as a result, the power of health authorities to effect change through the market mechanism. These constraints have been cited as key reasons for non-use of economic evidence[9–11] and suggest economics may have to develop methods more appropriate for the context in which the results may be used.

In summary, the current approach seems to be one of changing the problem to fit the solution,[51] of undertaking economic evaluation blind to the conditions in which the results have to be applied. The current approach ignores behavioural analyses of decision making that explain the way in which decision makers actually take decisions, how and what information is used, the objectives and values of key decision makers, and the incentives and constraints they face in making free and informed choice between alternative treatments.[30] It also means that the relevance and accuracy of economic information in the local contexts in which it needs to be applied is questionable.

The discussion of the behavioural analyses is not a counsel of despair for those involved in economic evaluation. Indeed, there is scope here, as part of a strategy to promote the use of the results of economic evaluation, for economists to work with other disciplines to better understand and to help change incentives to encourage the use of research evidence.[52] However, the behavioural analyses do underline the need to consider, firstly, ways in which methods of economic evaluation can be improved to make information more relevant and accurate in a local context and, secondly, how economic information might be presented to decision makers, given the way in which information is used in the decision making process. In the "complex and contested"[39] world of EBM, the quality of evidence is crucial, although behavioural analyses warn us not to have naive expectations about the degree and types of influence that economic evaluation might have over decisions.

In the remainder of this chapter we begin to address this agenda. We discuss the nature of the decisions faced by healthcare decision makers and suggest that the information to support these decisions offered by conventional approaches to economic evaluation can be of limited value. In the next section we concentrate specifically on cost issues. Towards the end of the chapter we consider alternative approaches to economic evaluation.

Cost considerations in practice

The issue of the validity of cost data in practice has been extensively discussed in the literature on standards in economic evaluation.[6,7] Discussion has focussed on technical aspects of the production of the service in question or variations in the costs of inputs, such as hours of medical time, number of days of inpatient stay or type and dose of medication. Such problems may be adequately addressed using sensitivity analysis.[53] However, there are other potentially more important issues such as whether the resources required to produce a given service increase in direct proportion to the number of individuals treated, the extent to which opportunity costs are context-specific, and the extent to which decision makers accept that resources are fixed. We begin by discussing the issue of a "fixed budget".

Context, opportunity cost and the assumption of a fixed budget

Even though the principle of scarcity may be accepted, the assumption of a universal fixed budget does not necessarily hold because, as Sheldon and Maynard[54] emphasise, negotiation over budgets takes place at many levels, from inter-speciality negotiation within trusts to "bargaining" between public and government through the voting process. Players in these bargaining games are aware of the *elasticity* of solutions and their ability to influence the size of the budget. Some "successes" in securing increases in resources may be high profile, such as additional funds for winter crises in emergency admissions, waiting list initiatives and new service developments. The effect of these successes may be to undermine people's acceptance that resources are fixed. For example, attempts to apply lower-level constraints did little to convince GPs that their budgets were "fixed".[55] Negotiated agreements regarding levels of funding may be particularly sensitive to evidence of unmet demand from which individuals could clearly benefit.

An analogy can be made with the consumption choices facing parents where "need" may be represented by the number of children in the household.[56] A bundle of commodities will be purchased to maximise the welfare of the household within the budget constraint. With the addition of a further child, the budget constraint would inevitably become tighter, but

183

the additional "needs" of the household are likely to provoke a labour-supply response which will also change the budget constraint.[57] Whilst there is obviously an upper limit on feasible resources (there is a limit to the number of hours an individual can work in a day), budgets can be increased within this limit. In a similar way, a more accurate description of healthcare constraints might be that they are variable but inelastic. If this is the perception in the general population, it may be accepted that there is a need for accountability and frugality but that resources should be reallocated if budgets become too tight. This may explain the reluctance of the public to comply with prioritisation of activities between competing populations on the basis of cost when there is clear "need" established for both groups.[34]

It may also partially explain why healthcare professionals may be unwilling to adopt the population perspective. They might, in principle, share the aim of maximising the population's health. However, the maximisation of health in the area of decision making over which they exert control, that is, *their* patients, can conflict with maximisation of the population's health, and although the medical profession's own ethical code refers to scarcity and the need to use resources efficiently, it also states that this duty is subordinate to the professional duty to the individual who seeks his or her clinical advice.[58] In practice, therefore, when faced by individual patients, clinicians are likely to feel that managing the system-level resource constraint to the benefit of society as a whole is not their responsibility.

At a sub-system level, it is inevitable that the slackness of constraints will vary enormously between clinicians' areas of responsibility. The resultant variations in unused budgets are themselves a source of inefficiency relative to a "first-best" world in which money could be moved freely between budgets. In an ideal world, economic evaluations taken from a societal perspective should not reflect these rigidities. Rather, policy makers should change the budget mechanism to ensure the optimal solution is feasible. However, these budgetary boundaries are a reality of the actual decision making process. Economic evaluations which rest on the principle of a universal budget constraint binding all decision makers equally may prescribe the optimal allocation in a first-best world but may suggest options which are neither feasible in practice due to budget rigidities nor efficient given that these rigidities exist.

A second problem relates to the inferences that can be drawn from cost data originating in this "second-best" world. Such measures of resources used in the provision of a service do not provide an accurate measure of the opportunity costs faced by the individual decision maker. In practice it may not be clear that resources have a foregone next-best use when the redeployment of resources is not feasible. As a consequence, the "prices" which have been attached to those units of resources do not reflect opportunity costs in the eyes of the decision maker. In the absence of perfectly flexible budgets, we may observe resource utilisation which is not

184

optimal in the long-run societal sense, but is "second-best" given the limited range of alternative uses of resources open to the decision maker.

Economies of scale and scope in practice

At the hospital level, it has been observed that costs and the number of people treated do not increase in direct proportion to each other.[59,60] It is likely that this is also true for the delivery of specific services within hospitals. Moreover learning, which is a clinician/service phenomenon, is a determinant of both outcome and cost.[60–62] On the benefit side, if individuals are prioritised on the basis of capacity to benefit, benefits per patient will decline as more patients are treated. Interdependence between the costs of different programmes (economies of scope), because various programmes can draw on common facilities or resources, have also been found at the hospital level.[59]

The importance of local circumstances

Bryan and Brown[63] have highlighted the importance of local circumstances for considerations of cost-effectiveness. They suggested that local circumstances may be important for three reasons:

- Local unit-costs may differ from national unit-costs
- Local unit-benefits may differ from national unit-benefits
- The alternatives may differ locally from the alternatives considered in published studies.

The implications of the first two of these three considerations for local cost-effectiveness considerations are relatively straightforward. The last consideration is more difficult to interpret but can be shown with a simple example. The example is hypothetical but demonstrates first, the potential problems of using unit-costs and second, the importance of local circumstances.

For our example, we consider the type of decision that might be faced in a general practice regarding the best way to use the resources at its disposal to increase the quality of care it provides. Assume that the practice wishes to maximise the "enablement" of its patients on the grounds that patients' feelings and perceptions about life are an important predictor of outcome. Enablement has been measured using the Patient Enablement Instrument which assesses the extent to which people feel they are better able, as result of visiting their doctor, to cope with life, to understand and cope with their illness, to keep themselves healthy and to help themselves. It also asks whether people feel more confident about their health after visiting their doctor.[64]

Imagine that it is known that General Practitioners provide 20 hours of patient contact time per week at a total cost of £800. On average, they see 120 patients a week and produce an average enablement score of 3 in the patients that they see. They therefore generate 18 "units of patient enablement" (UPEs) per hour. Also imagine that practice nurses provide 20 hours of patient contact time per week at a total cost of £400. On average, they see 80 patients per week and produce an average enablement score of 1·5 in the patients that they see. They therefore generate 6 UPEs per hour. In summary, the average costs and benefits of GPs are 18 UPEs per hour for £40 and of practice nurses are 6 UPEs per hour for £20.

A particular general practice is considering whether to introduce a new intervention that can be delivered in two different ways. The first method involves five hours of GP time, at an implied cost of £200, and produces 150 UPEs. The second method involves two-and-a-half hours of GP time and six hours of practice nurse time, at an implied cost of £220, and also produces 150 UPEs. Under these scenarios, the first method is a cheaper way of producing the same level of benefit and is the recommended option.

However, if we consider the choice in terms of opportunity costs rather than financial costs, we find that the first method, involving five hours of GP time, is equivalent to 90 UPEs foregone. On the other hand, the second method, involving two-and-a-half hours of GP time and six hours of practice nurse time, is equivalent to 81 UPEs foregone. Therefore, because unit-costs do not reflect the "value" of different inputs, the second method is actually the recommended option.

However, in this particular practice, routine activity by practice nurses is discovered, perhaps by audit, to be more productive than the average, say 12 UPEs per hour. This may be because the client groups are different locally so that, for example, there are more patients with psychological problems in whom higher UPE scores are achieved. Alternatively, it may be because practice nurses are more scarce, and therefore their current activity is more valuable in the sense that their existing workload is limited to a smaller number of patients in whom the benefits of treatment are greater. The differences may also arise because the practice offers a triage system for first contacts. Whatever the reason(s), the opportunity costs are different locally and, while the first method represents 90 UPEs foregone as before, the second method now represents 117 UPEs foregone. Under this scenario, the first method is again the preferred option.

While this is clearly an abstract and hypothetical example, it does demonstrate that use of unit-costs can be misleading and that local conditions are relevant when considering the evidence on cost-effectiveness. It is also important to note that the importance of local conditions has been demonstrated without introducing local variation in either unit-costs or unit-benefits from the possible interventions being compared. These would introduce additional relevant local considerations.

186

Coast et al.[65] have also highlighted that local implementation issues can have a profound effect on the cost-effectiveness of different options. Drawing together several published studies of hospital-at-home versus hospital care, they consider how the cost-effectiveness of hospital-at-home will depend on how much activity is transferred out of hospital and how the transfer of activity is funded. Small transfers of activity out of hospital permit only limited amounts of resources to be released since a large proportion of hospital resources are fixed financial commitments. Similarly, without a transfer of resources out of hospital, the cost-effectiveness of hospital-at-home will depend on how the released resources within the hospital sector are used and what activities in the community sector must be displaced to provide hospital-at-home care.

The potential problems with cost data are often discussed in abstract terms and of course their importance will depend on the extent to which they occur in practice. Much of the work on evaluating medical interventions from an economic perspective has taken place on pharmaceuticals. These interventions may have quite uniform unit-costs and may not become cheaper as more individuals are treated. Moreover they may be more likely to come from a common budget and it may be possible to switch resources between alternatives quite easily. However, interventions that require capital goods such as equipment become cheaper per person treated as number of individuals treated expands.

It is perhaps labour inputs which are of particular interest. The amount of resource available is likely to be quite flexible as "effort" can be manipulated and will respond to "demand". Therefore, it is likely that there will be increasing returns to scale in numbers treated although this may be offset by decreasing returns to scale in quality. We may also expect problems in switching these resources across different budget boundaries.

Alternative options for promoting economic considerations in practice

Opportunity costs are context-specific because they are related to the available budget and the range of feasible local alternatives being evaluated.[66] To assess whether estimated costs can be generalised to other contexts it has been proposed that, in addition to an overall cost figure, input requirements for evaluated alternatives be presented in disaggregated form.[7,67] However, this still does not take account of stepped relationships between costs and the number of patients treated.

Therefore, to reflect opportunity cost more accurately, Birch et al.[66] propose a three-stage approach to evaluating proposed changes:

187

1 Evaluate the expected additional benefits from the proposed change
2 Identify the resources needed and where they are likely to come from
3 Estimate the benefits which would be lost from stopping these activities.

This requires a fundamentally different design to the standard method of allocating equal numbers to different treatments and then counting the costs of production and the benefits. In this section we discuss an alternative method of constructing a trial which implements this framework by holding opportunity costs constant.

These proposed designs are examples of one of the few options proposed by Birch and Gafni[3] for ensuring cost-effectiveness studies are compatible with welfare economics. In these designs the aim is to express opportunity costs in non-monetary terms. The idea of expressing opportunity costs in non-monetary terms is not new. In a series of applications, Torgerson and colleagues have indicated how many more individuals could have received treatment if relatively costly service options were not adopted.[68-70]

Studies of proposed changes to health care delivery include some or all of the following considerations: different interventions (for example group counselling or individual interviews); different inputs (for example General Practitioners or practice nurses); and/or different populations, perhaps defined on the basis of age groups. To simplify the exposition we consider three possible types of comparisons:

1 A comparison of different interventions delivered by the same inputs to the same population.
2 A comparison of the same intervention delivered by the same inputs on different populations.
3 A comparison of the same intervention delivered by different inputs on the same population.

1 Different interventions delivered by the same inputs to the same population

The basic approach to comparisons of this type is to allocate equal levels of resources to each programme in the study. Sutton shows how such a cost-constrained design might look in practice by considering a hypothetical example of a brief versus more intensive intervention for alcoholism.[71] This example, which uses effectiveness figures produced by Chapman and Huygens,[72] is reproduced in Table 15.1. Although the brief intervention is no more effective per person than the intensive intervention, it produces successful outcomes for many more individuals (16 v 3). Therefore, the opportunity costs of allocating 1·5 full-time equivalent workers to the intensive intervention are readily seen in the outcome figures.

188

Table 15.1 Hypothetical cost-constrained study of a brief versus more intensive intervention for alcoholism.

Programme	Staff-time (full-time equivalent)	Estimated number of subjects treated	Rate of problem-free drinking (%)[c]	Number of problem-free drinkers
Outpatient	1·5	10[a]	28·6	3
Confrontational interview	1·5	72[b]	22·2	16

Taken from Sutton.[71] Original effectiveness figures taken from Chapman and Huygens[72]

a Based on twice-weekly sessions for 2 groups of 5 subjects run by a multi-disciplinary team of 3 half-time workers over a 6-week period.
b Based on two-hourly sessions at a rate of 1 each per day for 4 days per week by 3 half-time workers over a 6-week period.
c Source: Chapman and Huygens.[72]

This cost-constrained design has several potentially useful features. Firstly, it more directly relates to the problem of achieving the most health outcome from a fixed budget. Secondly, by comparing alternatives at a given input level, it allows for partial or full indivisibility and increasing or decreasing returns to scale. Of course, the problem of generalisability of a production function from a certain setting remains, as does the possibility of economies of scope. Multi-site studies would help in this regard.[53]

In addition this approach makes a number of assumptions in making cost-effectiveness ratios rather more explicit. The higher per person resource requirements of some interventions become apparent because less people can be treated and the trade-off between quantity and quality is no longer hidden in the cost-effectiveness ratio. By specifying the resources used in the cost-constrained design, comparisons across studies are still possible.

The study design is likely to result in different numbers of patients being treated in each arm of the trial. This unequal randomisation will increase the statistical power of the study since more patients are allocated to the less costly intervention.[73] Sutton shows that if ethics are extended to those who miss out on receiving treatment because of the resources used (i.e. those who bear the opportunity cost), there are no additional ethical problems with exposing different numbers of patients *ex ante* to treatments which may be of different effectiveness *ex post*.[71,73]

A cost-constrained design may also reduce the amount of involvement needed from economists. In some situations it may only be necessary to consider the major components of cost. Evaluations may be able to proceed without detailed cost analysis, even though the resultant analyses would be partial on the cost side. With its provider-based focus, this might encourage clinicians to become involved in economic evaluations.[14]

2 The same intervention delivered by the same inputs to different populations

Torgerson and colleagues provide examples of this type of comparison.[68-70] Because such comparisons are based on reallocation *within* the relevant budget, they cannot be compared with policy changes involving shifts in resources across budgets. One of the studies considers changing the age-group to which breast-cancer screening is targeted and indicates greater effectiveness of screening older age-groups.[69] Fundamentally, the decision depends on the importance attached to treating different groups of the population.

3 The same intervention delivered by different inputs to the same population

The third possible comparison is the most difficult to evaluate without recourse to cost information. For example, we may wish to compare the cost-effectiveness of intervention delivered by either a hospital consultant or a general practitioner. The traditional approach would be to value each staff input at its wage rate. This implies an opportunity cost of time equal to the wage rate which is only justifiable in terms of a perfectly competitive labour market.

In practice we would want to identify what activities would be displaced for the GP and taken up by the consultant. The changing demands on the consultant and GP may only provoke corresponding labour-supply responses (i.e. the consultant works slightly less hours and the GP slightly more) or changes in the quality of services for other patients. The problem is essentially that the traditional study design does not fully answer the question, since the proposed change of work for the consultant should be evaluated alongside the proposed change of work for the GP. The appropriate design for this type of comparison should be to identify the *full* implications of the proposed change for the *total* benefit produced by those inputs.

Extending the definition of acceptable evidence and the type of evidence used

We have suggested that economic evaluation techniques, and particularly the treatment of opportunity costs, are highly simplistic and could give rise to misleading recommendations. This simplicity has probably arisen because economic evaluations have been linked to RCTs and economic evaluation methodology has become rather isolated from mainstream economics. Economists have developed a substantial body of theoretical

190

and empirical work explaining, *inter alia*, the impact of health care on health relative to the influence of other factors such as "lifestyle", environment, deprivation and education, or the factors influencing clinicians' behaviour with respect to levels or combinations of care delivered. However, the evaluation literature has developed almost in isolation from other economic analyses of health and health care. For example, this wider economic literature would not support the assumptions that one of the main resource inputs to primary care (GP time) is fixed[74] or that slack hospital resources can be easily reallocated.[75] Therefore, if we cannot identify the alternative use of the resources, or if we want to allow for changes in the overall size of the budget (for example labour-supply response), slackness in the resource constraint or a flexible cost-quality relationship, we may need to rely on behavioural models of decision makers and analyses of observational data.

Outside of the health field, an experimental approach is relatively alien to economists who rely mainly on analysis of secondary, observational data sources.[76] The problems of confounding have dissuaded many from relying on observational data for estimates of treatment effects, and economic evaluations have been criticised for utilising these data.[77,78] However, recently there have been considerable advances in the methods for controlling confounding,[79] and discussion of the advantages of the treatment effects which are estimated.[80] Analysis of observational data offers the possibility of investigating effects otherwise not perceptible, such as macro-level effects[81] and unobservable patient benefits.[82] Increased application of these techniques would be a suitable complement to the recent moves towards increasingly pragmatic trials.

Conclusion

Other chapters have presented a variety of reasons for variations in the uptake of evidence on the effectiveness of clinical practice. The implementation of findings from economic analyses raises additional issues. In this chapter, particular problems associated with the application of economics information have been highlighted.

Encouraging implementation of economic findings is not simply a matter of providing more and better-quality economic evidence. Establishing standardised methods for economic evaluations[6-8] may actually delay implementation if there is reaction from the supply-side, such that researchers who are potentially interested in the principles of cost-effectiveness are deterred from becoming involved. The promotion of standardised methods must go hand in hand with increases in the capacity of the research community to conduct and understand studies using these methods.

However, in this chapter, whilst welcoming the efforts to promote such methods, we have questioned the impact evaluations based on these methods are likely to have, firstly, because of the nature of the decision making process, and secondly, because these methods may not be relevant to or accurate in the context in which the results are used. Decision makers may not (think they) face fixed budgets. They may face alternative uses of resources which are not perfectly divisible in terms of either costs or benefits, or which are not feasible locally. In addition, they may have objectives which are not coincident with the particular social goals specified in economic evaluations. As noted above, in the long-term the former could be tackled by increasing the flexibility of budget allocations, the latter by changing the incentive structure. Whilst implementation of service changes preferred from the societal perspective should remain the long-term goal, there are a number of other options for encouraging the use of economic evaluation in the short-term by modifying the methods used to more accurately reflect local opportunity costs.

Locally relevant and accurate economic evaluation requires three steps: estimation of the benefits of implementing the proposed programme; identification of the resources required to implement the proposed changes and where they are to be obtained from; and estimation of the loss in benefits from the original source of funds.

The traditional approach of conducting economic evaluations alongside clinical trials leaves local cost considerations as an afterthought. In this chapter we have discussed study designs which place the actual opportunity costs faced by decision makers at the centre of the analysis. We have also proposed that analyses should be conducted based on a range of objectives which decision makers may want to maximise. This range of alternatives could be inferred from analysis of actual behaviour or trials based on what we believe are decision makers' objectives. We believe that by focusing more clearly on the nature of the "real-life" decision and the reason *why* cost considerations are pertinent, this approach may encourage greater participation of providers in evaluation and the use of the results of economic evaluation.

Improvement of the information upon which the choices are made is necessary but not sufficient to ensure an effective role for economics in the prioritisation of healthcare resources. Priority setting is a complex process of choice. Consideration should be given by those using economic evaluations to the processes by which choices are actually made, by whom, to what end and under what constraints. Together with the methodological development of economic evaluation using pragmatic study designs and observational data where appropriate, this would help to ensure greater implementation of economic recommendations.

Acknowledgements

We are grateful for helpful comments on previous options by the editors, an anonymous referee and several colleagues, including Steve Birch, Diane Dawson, Martin Roland and Trevor Sheldon. Matt Sutton is funded by the University of Glasgow and the Information and Statistics Division of the Common Services Agency of the NHSiS. The usual disclaimers apply.

References

1 Haynes B, Haines A. Barriers and bridges to evidence based practice. In Haines A, Donald A, eds. *Getting Research into Practice*. London: BMJ Publishing, 1998.
2 Phelps CE, Mushlin AI. On the (near) equivalence of cost effectiveness and cost benefit analysis. *Int J Tech Assess Health Care* 1991;7:12–21.
3 Birch S, Gafni A. Cost effectiveness/utility analyses. Do current decision rules lead us to where we want to be? *J Health Econ* 1992;11:279–96.
4 Pauly MV. Valuing health benefits in money terms. In Sloan FA, ed. *Valuing Health Care: Costs Benefits and Effectiveness of Pharmaceuticals and Other Medical Technologies*. Cambridge: Cambridge University Press, 1995.
5 Garber AM, Phelps CE. Economic foundations of cost-effectiveness analysis. *Health Econ* 1997;16:1–31.
6 Weinstein MC, Siegel JE, Gold MR, Kamlet MS, Russell LB. Recommendations of the panel on cost-effectiveness in health and medicine. *JAMA* 1996;276:1253–8.
7 Drummond MF, Jefferson T. Guidelines for authors and peer reviewers of economic submissions to the BMJ. *BMJ* 1996;313:275–83.
8 Sheldon TA, Vanoli A. Providing research intelligence to the NHS: the role of the NHS Centre for Reviews and Dissemination. In Towse A, ed. *Guidelines for the Economic Evaluation of Pharmaceuticals: Can the UK learn from Australia and Canada?* London: OHE, 1997.
9 Drummond M, Cooke J, Walley J. Economic evaluation under managed competition: evidence from the UK. *Soc Sci Med* 1997;45:583–5.
10 Duthie T, Trueman P, Chancellor J, Diez L. Research into the use of health economics in decision making in the United Kingdom – Phase II. Is health economics 'for good or evil'? *Health Policy* 1999;46:143–57.
11 Crump B, Drummond M, Alexander S, Devaney C. Economic Evaluation in the United Kingdom National Health Service. In Graf von der Schulenberg JM, ed. *The Influence of Economic Evaluation Studies on Health Care Decision Making*. IOS Press, 2000.
12 Reinhardt U. Making economic evaluations respectable. *Soc Sci Med* 1997;45:555–62.
13 Williams A. How should information on cost effectiveness influence clinical practice? In Delamothe T, ed. *Outcomes into clinical practice*, pp 99–107. London: BMJ Publishing Group, 1994.
14 Dowie J. Clinical trials *and* economic evaluations? No, there are only evaluations. *Health Econ* 1997;6:87–9.
15 Sloan FA, ed. *Valuing Health Care: Costs Benefits and Effectiveness of Pharmaceuticals and Other Medical Technologies*. Cambridge: Cambridge University Press, 1995.
16 Drummond MF, O'Brien B, Stoddart GS, Torrance GW. *Methods for the Economic Evaluation of Health Care Programmes*. Oxford: Oxford University Press, 1997.
17 Drummond MF, Mason J. Reporting guidelines for economic studies [editorial]. *Health Econ* 1995;4:85–94.
18 Briggs A, Sculpher M. Sensitivity analysis in economic evaluation: a review of published studies. *Health Econ* 1995;4:355–72.
19 Williams A. Economics, society and health care ethics. In Gillon R, ed. *Principles of health care ethics*, pp 829–42. Chichester: Wiley, 1994.

20 Weinstein MC, Zeckhauser R. Critical ratios and efficient allocation. *J Public Econ* 1973;**2**:147–57.

21 Johanesson M. A note on the depreciation of the societal perspective in economic evaluation of health care. *Health Policy* 1995;**33**:59–66.

22 Mishan EJ. *Cost benefit analysis.* Massachusetts: Unwin Hyman Ltd, 1988.

23 Ryan M, Shackley P. Assessing the benefits of health care: how far should we go? *Qual Health Care* 1995;**4**:207–13.

24 Sugden R, Williams A. *The principles of practical cost-benefit analysis.* Oxford: Oxford University Press, 1978.

25 Culyer AJ. The normative economics of health care finance and provision. *Ox Rev Econ Policy* 1989;**5**:34–58.

26 Knapp M, Beecham J, Anderson J *et al.* The TAPS Project. 3: Predicting the Community Costs of Closing Psychiatric Hospitals. *Br J Psychiatry* 1990;**157**:661–70.

27 Torgerson DJ, Spencer A. Marginal costs and benefits. *BMJ* 1996;**312**:35–6.

28 Birch S, Gafni A. Cost-effectiveness ratios: in a league of their own. *Health Policy* 1994;**28**:133–41.

29 Stinnett AA, Paltiel AD. Mathematical programming for the efficient allocation of health care resources. *J Health Econ* 1996;**15**:641–53.

30 Harrison S. The politics of evidence-based medicine in the United Kingdom. *Policy and Politics* 1998;**26**:15–31.

31 Scottish Office Department of Health. *Towards a Healthier Scotland: A White Paper on Health.* Edinburgh: The Stationery Office, 1999.

32 NHS Executive. *Changing the Internal Market: EL(97)33.* Leeds: Department of Health, 1997.

33 Rosen R. Applying research to health care policy and practice: medical and managerial views on effectiveness and the role of research. *J Health Serv Res Policy* 2000;**5**:103–8.

34 Nord E, Richardson J, Street A, Kuhse H, Singer P. Who cares about cost? Does economic analysis impose or reflect social values? *Health Policy* 1995;**34**:79–94.

35 Abel Olsen J, Donaldson C. Helicopters, hearts and hips: using willingness to pay to set priorities for public sector health care programmes. *Soc Sci and Med* 1998;**46**:1–12.

36 Nord E. The trade off between severity of illness and treatment effect in cost-value analysis of health care. *Health Policy* 1993;**24**:227–38.

37 Tengs TO. An evaluation of Oregon's Medicaid rationing algorithms. *Health Econ* 1996;**5**:171–81.

38 Hadorn D. The Oregon priority-setting exercise: cost-effectiveness and the rule of rescue, revisited. *Med Decis Making* 1996;**16**:117–19.

39 Ferlie E, Fitzgerald L, Wood M. Getting evidence into clinical practice: an organisational behaviour perspective. *J Health Serv Res Policy* 2000;**5**:96–102.

40 Mooney G, Ryan M. Agency in health care – getting beyond first principles. *J Health Econ* 1993;**12**:125–35.

41 Elliott H, Popay J. How are policy makers using evidence? Models of research utilisation and local NHS policy making. *J Epidemiol Community Health* 2000;**54**:461–8.

42 Whynes DK. Towards an evidence-based National Health Service? *Economic J* 1996;**106**:1702–12.

43 Escarce JJ. Externalities in hospitals and physician adoption of a new surgical technology: An exploratory analysis. *J Health Econ* 1996;**15**:715–34.

44 Hirshleifer D. The blind leading the blind. Social influence, fads and informational cascades. In Tomassi M, Ierulli K, eds. *The New Economics of Human Behaviour.* Cambridge: Cambridge University Press, 1995.

45 Drummond MF, Aristides M. The Australian cost-effectiveness guidelines: an update. In Towse A, ed. *Guidelines for the Economic Evaluation of Pharmaceuticals: Can the UK Learn from Australia and Canada?* London: OHE, 1997.

46 Culyer AJ, Posnett J. Hospital behaviour and competition. In Culyer AJ, Maynard A, Posnett J, eds. *Competition in Health Care: Reforming the NHS,* pp 12–47. Basingstoke: Macmillan, 1990.

47 Robinson R. The impact of the NHS reforms 1991–1995: a review of research evidence. *J Pub Health Med* 1996;**18**:337–42.

48 LeGrand J, Mays N, Mulligan J. *Learning from the NHS Internal Market: A review of the evidence*. London: King's Fund, 1998.
49 Chalkley M, Malcolmson J. Contracts for the National Health Service. *Economic J* 1996;**106**:1691–701.
50 Propper C, Bartlett W. The impact of competition on the behaviour of National Health Service trusts. In Flynn R, Williams G, eds. *Contracting for Health: Quasi-Markets and the NHS*. Oxford: Oxford University Press, 1997.
51 Birch S, Gafni A. Changing the problem to fit the solution: Johanneson and Weinstein's (mis) application of economics to real world problems. *J Health Econ* 1993;**12**:469–76.
52 Maynard A, Kanavos P. Health economics: an evolving paradigm. *Health Econ* 2000;**9**:183–90.
53 Briggs A, Sculpher M, Buxton MJ. Uncertainty in the economic evaluation of health care technologies: the role of sensitivity analysis. *Health Econ* 1994;**3**:95–104.
54 Sheldon TA, Maynard A. Is rationing inevitable? In: *Rationing in Action*. London: BMJ Publishing Group, 1993.
55 Scott A, Wordsworth S, Donaldson C. *Using economics in a primary care led NHS: applying PBMA to GP Fundholding*. Paper presented to Health Economists' Study Group, Brunel University, 1996.
56 Browning M. Children and household economic behaviour. *J Econ Lit* 1992;**30**:1434–75.
57 Browning M, Deaton A, Irish M. A profitable approach to labour supply and commodity demands over the life-cycle. *Econometrica* 1985;**53**:503–43.
58 British Medical Association. *The Handbook of Medical Ethics*. London: British Medical Association, 1984.
59 Butler JRG. *Hospital Cost Analysis*. London: Kluwer Academic Publishers, 1995.
60 Centre for Reviews and Dissemination. *Hospital volume and health care outcomes, costs and patient access*. Bulletin 2(8). York: NHSCRD, 1996.
61 Hamilton BH, Hamilton VH. Estimating surgical volume-outcome relationships applying survival models: accounting for frailty and hospital fixed effects. *Health Econ* 1997;**6**:383–96.
62 Langkilde LK, Sogaard J. The adjustment of cost measurement to account for learning. *Health Econ* 1997;**6**:83–6.
63 Bryan S, Brown J. Extrapolation of cost-effectiveness information to local settings. *J Health Serv Res Policy* 1998;**3**:108–12.
64 Howie JGR, Heaney DJ, Maxell M, Walker JJ, Freeman GK, Rai H. Quality at general practice consultations: cross-sectional survey. *BMJ* 1999;**319**:738–43.
65 Coast J, Hensher M, Mulligan J, Shepperd S, Jones J. Conceptual and practical difficulties with the economic evaluation of health service developments. *J Health Serv Res Policy* 2000;**5**:42–8.
66 Birch S, Leake JL, Lewis DW. Economic issues in the development and use of practice guidelines: an application to resource allocation in dentistry. *Community Dent Health* 1996;**13**:70–5.
67 Walker A, Major K, Young D, Brown A. *Economic costs in the NHS: A useful insight or just bad accountancy?* Paper presented to the Health Economists' Study Group, Liverpool University, 1997.
68 Torgerson DJ, Donaldson C, Garton MJ, Reid DM, Russell IT. Recruitment methods for screening programmes: the price of high compliance. *Health Econ* 1993;**2**:55–8.
69 Torgerson DJ, Gosden T. The National Breast Screening service: is it economically efficient? *Q J Med* 1997;**90**:423–5.
70 Torgerson DJ, Donaldson C. An economic view of high compliance as a screening objective. *BMJ* 1994;**308**:117–19.
71 Sutton M. Personal paper: how to get the best health outcome from given amount of money. *BMJ* 1997;**315**:47–19.
72 Chapman PLH, Huygens I. An evaluation of three treatment programmes for alcoholism: an experimental study with 6- and 18-month follow-ups. *Br J Addict* 1988;**83**:67–81.
73 Torgerson DJ, Campbell M. Unequal randomisation can improve the economic efficiency of clinical trials. *J Health Serv Res Policy* 1997;**2**:81–5.
74 Scott A, Hall J. Evaluating the effects of GP remuneration: problems and prospects. *Health Policy* 1995;**31**:183–95.

75 Hughes D, McGuire A. *An Empirical Investigation of Hospital Cost Functions Introducing Output Heterogeneity and Controlling for Demand Uncertainty*. Paper presented to Health Economists' Study Group, University of York, 1997.

76 Hey J. *Experiments in Economics*. Oxford: Blackwell, 1992.

77 Sheldon TA. Problems of using modelling in the economic evaluation of health care. *Health Econ* 1996;5:1–11.

78 Buxton MJ, Drummond MF, van Hout BA *et al*. Modelling in economic evaluation: an unavoidable fact of life. *Health Econ* 1997;6:217–27.

79 McClellan M, McNeill BJ, Newhouse JP. Does more intensive treatment of acute myocardial patients in the elderly reduce mortality: analysis using instrumental variables. *JAMA* 1994;272:859–66.

80 Heckman JJ. Instrumental variables: a study of implicit behavioral assumptions used in making program evaluations. *J Hum Resour* 1997;32:441–61.

81 Garfinkel I, Manski CF, Michalopoulus C. Micro experiments and macro effects. In Manski CF, Garfinkel I, eds. *Evaluating Welfare and Training Programs*. Cambridge: Harvard University Press, 1992.

82 Philipson T, Hedges LV. Treatment evaluation through social experiments: subjects vs. investigators. Mimeo. Chicago: Department of Economics, University of Chicago, 1996.

83 Weinstein MC. From cost-effectiveness ratios to resource allocation: where to draw the line? In Sloan FA, ed. *Valuing Health Care: Costs Benefits and Effectiveness of Pharmaceuticals and Other Medical Technologies*. Cambridge: Cambridge University Press, 1995.

16 Surviving research implementation

DAVID EVANS AND LESLEY WYE

Key messages

- A key to surviving research implementation is in the change facilitator's ability to simultaneously manage many inherent tensions including:

  - Keeping the project modest and deliverable while justifying the expense and effort required to make even small changes.
  - Buliding up good relationships with a wide variety of key individuals and planning the process appropriately while achieving enough "early wins" to sustain interest.
  - Recognising the limitations of evidence as a tool for fostering change while promoting an "evidence-based" culture.
  - Working towards embedding change within the system (which necessarily means eliminating the change facilitator's role) while maintaining enthusiasm for the project over a long period of time.

- Good change facilitators are a precious resource and further support for them and their work is needed to help ensure that we reap the full benefits of health research.

Introduction

This chapter is included primarily as an aid to those who are inspired, perhaps by other chapters in this book, to set out to implement changes in their own workplaces based on research evidence. It reflects the reality of experience in one corner of the UK's NHS, reminding us that what appears to be simple usually turns out to be complicated, and that the quality of communication may be equally as important as the quality of evidence.

What follows is based on the cumulative experienwce of more than 22 people who led research implementation projects in a broad cross-section of NHS contexts in one NHS region (North Thames) over a two-year period (1996–1998)(see Table 16.1). It draws on their candid accounts of the successes and failures they experienced,[1] from an external evaluation of the projects,[2] and a series of follow-up interviews with a sub-set of nine project

Table 16.1 The North Thames Health Authority-led R&D implementation projects.

Health Authority	Subject of Research and Development implementation project(s)
Barking & Havering	Coronary heart disease, and obstetrics and gynaecology
Barnet	Back pain; diabetic retinopathy; *H. pylori*
Brent & Harrow	Protocols in A&E
Brent & Harrow	Non-invasive cardiac assessment
Brent & Harrow	Schizophrenia (*did not start*)
Camden & Islington	*H. pylori* eradication
Ealing, Hammersmith and Hounslow	Diabetes register
East London and the City	Cardiac interventions
East London and the City	Leg ulcers
Enfield and Haringey	GP Learning Sets
Hillingdon	*H. pylori*; leg ulcers; congenital heart disease
Kensington, Chelsea and Westminster	Dyspepsia (*did not start*)
Kensington, Chelsea and Westminster	Echocardiography and ACE inhibitors
North Essex	Cancer services
Redbridge and Waltham Forest	Diabetes; asthma; hypertension
South Essex	Hypertension in the elderly
West Hertfordshire	Anticoagulation

team members. The authors were both involved with the projects as external observers, and we are greatly indebted to the project team members for their frank and generously given insights, upon which this work is based.

The differences and contradictions in the experiences of those who led the North Thames projects highlights the complexity of this type of activity, and shows the extent to which local context impacts upon implementation. This is not a "how to ..." guide, nor a series of checklists, both of which we consider to be of very limited help in these situations where flexibility, trust, and incremental advance fit much better than rigid formulas or pat "solutions". Resisting the temptation to present a simplistic blueprint, we have instead tried to identify tensions, which arise when taking on the challenging business of implementation. This chapter introduces the uncomfortable idea that the success of an implementation project and the well-being of those involved as change agents may not necessarily be mutually compatible. Where these interests diverge, our emphasis is on the experience of the individual, and our objective is to help those in similar situations to survive the experience.

Tension No. 1: Modest objectives and realistic boundaries vs. making a big enough difference

One theme that emerged consistently in the retrospective reflections of project team members in the North Thames research implementation projects was that of the need to keep objectives modest and manageable. In every one of the projects (17 in total), those involved had to a greater or lesser extent initially overestimated what it would be possible to achieve. For example, one project anticipated recruiting 80% of GPs in the Health Authority to the project and "supporting" 18 evidence-based initiatives. In another health authority, the project team expected that their implementation project would result in "evidence of effectiveness" being established as a guiding principle underpinning its commissioning activity. Not surprisingly, neither realised these ambitious objectives; nevertheless they did achieve some progress. In the first example, 25% of GPs were recruited to the project, and they reviewed the evidence for nine topics. In the second, evidence-based commissioning did not become a reality, but 17 GP practices became much more aware of evidence-based approaches to coronary heart disease through auditing the implementation of a set of guidelines.

With hindsight almost all of those involved in the North Thames projects wished that they had been less ambitious in their initial objectives. They acknowledged that important and sustainable changes are most likely to be achieved by a succession of small steps, rather than a leap. They wished that they had been more aware and willing to accept that relatively slow, incremental change could be worthwhile. As one project lead put it:

> I wanted it to be perfect. But I've learnt that big things can come from small things.

We consider the tension here to be between having modest, deliverable objectives yet being able to justify the expense and effort required, when the changes achieved may be criticised as being inconsequential. One local clinician summed up his frustration with the lack of appreciation for the length of time necessary to implement change commenting:

> It's the same problem with all evidence-based projects. They take a long time to set up and the money runs out just when it's about to take off and you can't show any benefit yet.

This professional, like others involved in the North Thames Health Authority-led implementation projects, has learned first hand the amount of energy needed to implement changes based on research evidence in the NHS. They appreciate that a small shift in the right direction is usually the best way to begin a bigger turn.

Tension No. 2: Laying the groundwork vs. achieving early successes

Successful implementation depends on gaining the respect and support of key individuals who have influence over others and access to the resources necessary to support change. Achieving visible early success may therefore be critical in establishing the viability of an implementation project (and ensuring that the change agent's contract is renewed to keep the project going).

Unfortunately, a major, though often hurried preliminary task is getting an understanding of the local context and relationship building, for which there are few measurable indicators. Change agents work towards ensuring that they have obtained and conveyed the right information to and from key individuals and that a critical mass of enthusiasts is established. One of the project leads from North Thames said that this had involved:

> ... identifying allies, listening and asking questions, observing and trying to get enough background information so I don't tread on someone else's toes. It's all about fact finding, gathering intelligence data and feeling my way.

During this crucial phase of the project, change agents help individuals move from a vague sense that something needs to be done, to a genuine commitment to implement change and onto concrete action. This usually takes much longer than initially estimated, and requires the involvement of enough of the key people at roughly the same time. What happens in this crucial phase is presented in a useful model developed by US psychologists Prochaska and di Clemente[3] as shown in Figure 16.1.

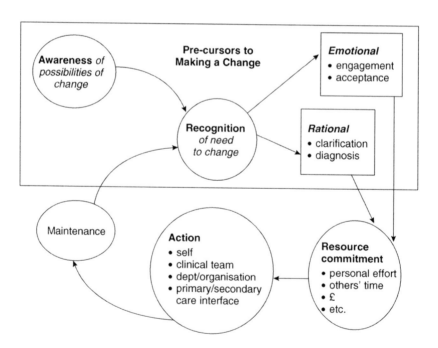

Figure 16.1 Model for laying the groundwork to implement change.

Facilitating key individuals in this process from awareness and recognition through to the more measurable "action" phase is one function of the change agent. A tension arises because this difficult task usually has to be accomplished *at the same time* as demonstrating worthwhile progress in terms of visible outputs (or an "early win"). Striking a balance between the probably invisible (but essential) groundwork and a physical manifestation of the value of the work is therefore an important, and highly context-specific challenge.

Another aspect to laying the groundwork is good planning. In our follow-up interviews, the lesson most commonly cited by those who participated in the North Thames projects was that they now think that more detailed planning would be a priority if they were to tackle similar work again. But this is difficult to do. As one project lead commented:

> You don't have time to think up a project plan because people are so focused on outcomes. Even now, I have to remind myself to plan. Half of it is really good planning.

In several of the North Thames projects, weaknesses at the planning stage led to omissions which seemed unimportant at the time, but which proved to be highly problematic later. For example, in one case, despite firmly believing that their work was having a positive effect, the project participants had no way of demonstrating that their efforts were making a difference. Paradoxically, it was this group's eagerness to get cracking with implementing changes in the service that led them to forgo completing a sufficiently thorough baseline audit.

With better planning, this type of mistake might be avoided; fairly obvious things likely to impact on implementation can be predicted and plans made accordingly. However in many cases those barriers, clear with hindsight, simply would not have been identifiable in advance. In these circumstances, as several of the North Thames project leads suggested, the capacity to adapt was key. It was also noted as a tension, as *fluidity* in implementation could seem somehow incongruent in a context inspired and underpinned by *solid* "evidence":

> We came to realise as the project evolved, that greater flexibility was a virtue, and would be a strength rather than a weakness. It is in this respect that the contrast between the rigorous, inflexible approach, which gives rise to the highest quality research evidence, and the flexible, pragmatic approach necessary for research implementation is most marked.

Tension No. 3: Evidence as a lever for (or obstacle to) change

A key criterion for funding of the North Thames Health Authority-led research implementation projects was that they were based on "robust" research evidence. The programme was underpinned by the apparently logical and widespread assumption that the strength of evidence should correlate with ease of implementing change. This assumption was borne out in one project where the project lead noted that when relating the work to some of the clinicians involved, discussing the high quality of the research evidence had been important in gaining their respect and confidence.[4] Interestingly, however, during the course of the project it became apparent that despite its quality, the *applicability* of the evidence to the context of the project was much more questionable. This was due to key differences between the groups from whom the research evidence was obtained (mostly American men under age 60, being treated in secondary care), and the patients for whom changes in care informed by that evidence was being implemented, (mostly English women over age 60, being treated in primary care).[1] With hindsight, an important lesson from that project was the realisation that the published literature did not contain all the answers. Nevertheless in this project, good quality evidence had been essential in gaining the interest and confidence of the clinicians involved.

Positive reaction to robust research evidence was not, however, universal. To our surprise in some cases good quality evidence had actually *de-motivated* clinicians. One local professional involved in drafting guidelines commented:

> … [the clinicians] give me flak because they [the guidelines] are gold standard rather than what could be done practically. It's turning GPs away rather than involving them.

In the majority of the North Thames projects, for the sake of survival, it was usually necessary to temper striving for excellence, and use of "gold standard" evidence, with a degree of compromise. For example in one case, where guidelines were being introduced, something short of the ideal was accommodated in two ways. Firstly, it was realised that "gold standard" evidence simply did not exist for all conditions, so a pragmatic decision was taken to incorporate the "best available" evidence into each set of guidelines. Secondly, it was recognised that notwithstanding the strenuous effort of those leading the project, changing the behaviour of *every single* healthcare professional involved would be unachieveable:

> There is always some variation. You can't have 100%. I'm happy with 80%. You need to be reasonable. This kind of work raises the standards overall, but some will still be poorer than others.

In this example, taking realistic views of both the contribution of the research literature and the limits to the malleability of colleagues' behaviour, gave the implementation project practical potential which was to a large extent realised. Achieving relative progress took precedence over ideal, but unattainable objectives.

Tension No. 4: Personal survival vs. project sustainability

For most of the North Thames projects, having a dedicated project worker had been absolutely critical in getting an implementation project off the ground. Implementation always involves interaction between people, and the communication of messages that have an impact on others' lives. Therefore the interpersonal skills of a project leader may be of equal (or greater) importance to/(than) understanding the scientific evidence underpinning proposed changes.

Finding someone who has the necessary blend of enthusiasm, credibility, and political realism is difficult. But when long-term sustainability through embedded change is also an objective, a further quality may be demanded, which for most people is counter-intuitive. This is the willingness to work, perhaps from day one, towards a vision of the future in which the project lead him or herself has no role. In other words, whilst maintaining enthusiasm for the project, credibility amongst key players and a realistic sense of what is achievable, the project worker whose aim is to achieve embedded change, must from the outset, be writing *themselves* out of the script.

In early 2000, a year to 18 months after North Thames funding for the projects had finished, we revisited nine leads from eight of the 17 project teams. One of our aims was to find out what had happened to them after North Thames funding finished. What we discovered was that two of the nine thrived on the experience and continue to extend their involvement as change agents (one remained within the original organisation whilst the other had left to do similar work elsewhere). Five had stopped doing this type of work altogether; two of whom had returned to the role they had been doing before the project (or gone "back in the box", as one person described it); two had left the organisation entirely and one had been promoted to a more strategic position. The final two were "burnt out", even though they continued to be employed as change agents within the same organisations. Although both had achieved a great deal, they felt disillusioned with their organisations and pessimistic with regard to their ability to have any further impact:

> I've had a very difficult few months. There's been lots of paperwork and I question what I'm doing … If I weren't doing a [further degree], I would have moved on.

Interestingly, we noted that there was no relationship between the success of the project in changing clinical practice with the condition of the change agent at the end of it. We spoke to one change agent from each of the three most successful projects. One is still thriving; another is "burnt out" and a third is somewhere in between. Because our sample is so small, and the variables considerable, it would be wrong to try to draw firm or generalisable conclusions about the differences between change agents who thrived and those who did not. However, the change agents themselves made several observations on what helped (or hindered) their ability to come through the project intact.

One striking characteristic of those who emerged optimistic was their ability to distance themselves from rejection:

> My husband says I'm a salesperson, but I only sell things I believe in. And I don't take it personally if I am rejected. It's easier when you work in a team because then you can handle those knocks easier. It's hard on an individual.

They saw every "no" as a challenge and an opportunity to think through a different approach. They could also see how their work made a difference. This contrasted with one of the "burnt out" leads who remarked that a lack of visible linkage between effort and results had been in part responsible for his disillusionment:

> Although small changes can lead to a big impact, you won't see it for a long time. It gets dispiriting because you don't get much of a feel for what's really happening.

Those who thrived took heart from the accumulation of small changes and from observing an immediate impact, however small. They also tapped into what people naturally did well, capitalizing on the strengths of individuals. One gave the following example:

> I try to make day to day changes. I look at the system and see how the system as a whole can be changed. For example ... I realized that doctors were not good enough at IT, but they were good at writing ... [they] write and tick boxes on protocols ... the receptionists pass the notes under the scanner. This way ... receptionists can do what they are good at [keeping patient notes up to date], doctors can do what they are good at ... and I get the data I need.

A more thorough and well-designed study may identify a comprehensive range of qualities and characteristics that mark out those who flourish doing this kind of work from those who do it competently for a while, but move on, exhausted. However the limitations of our data, the complexity of the issues and settings of the North Thames projects, and the absence of a prospective study design have made it possible at present only to make a few observations which raise a number of questions and possibilities. We hope that in future, opportunities will arise for these important issues to be investigated more fully and explained clearly.

204

Conclusion

Along with other similar research implementation initiatives such as PACE[5], FACTS[6], "Front Line"[7], and "The National R&D Programme on The Evaluation of Methods to Promote the Implementation of Research Findings"[8] the North Thames Health Authority-led implementation projects have begun to help us to understand the dynamics of implementing changes in health care based on research evidence. Our view is that the role of the individuals at the centre of this activity has emerged as a critical factor in getting research findings into practice. Our hope is that in addition to directing effort and resources at *obtaining* research evidence, the custodians of the NHS and other healthcare systems will recognise the pivotal role of change facilitators in enabling the *implementation* of evidence. They are a precious resource. Further enquiry, understanding, development and support for those involved in implementation will help to ensure that society reaps the benefits of health research.

---

*PACE is the acronym for a national programme entitled Promoting Action on Clinical Effectiveness, which was another initiative intended to support implementation projects based on research evidence. The programme is described in detail in the book by Dunning *et al.*[5]

†FACTS is the acronym for a project entitled Framework for Appropriate Care Throughout Sheffield, which involved implementing changes in primary care practice. The initiative is described in the report by Eve *et al.*[6]

††"Front Line" is an abbreviation for the Front Line Evidence Based Medicine project, which was another research implementation initiative in North Thames. Further details are contained in the project's final report.[7]

§"The National R&D Programme on The Evaluation of Methods to Promote the Implementation of Research Findings" was a national R&D initiative forming part of the NHS R&D Programme.

References

1 Evans D, Haines A, eds. *Implementing Evidence Based Changes in Health Care*. Abingdon: Radcliffe Medical Press, 2000.
2 Wye L, McClenahan J. *Getting Better with Evidence*. London: King's Fund, 2000.
3 Prochaska J, DiClemente C. *The Trans-Theoretical approach*. London: Krieger Publishing, 1984.
4 Evans D, Hood S, Taylor S. Clinical effectiveness in the real world: lessons learned from a project to improve the management of patients with heart failure. *Clinical Governance Bulletin*, Vol. 1 No. 3. RSM Press, Dec 2000.
5 Dunning M, Abi-Aad G, Gilbert D, Hutton H, Brown C. *Experience, Evidence and Everyday Practice*. London: King's Fund, 1998.
6 Eve R, Golton I, Hodgkin P, Munro J, Musson G. *Learning from FACTS – Lessons from the framework for appropriate care throughout Sheffield (FACTS) project*. Occasional Paper No. 97/3. SCHARR, University of Sheffield, Sheffield 1997.
7 Donald A. *The Front Line Evidence-Based Medicine Project*, Final Report. NHS Executive (North Thames) 1998.
8 *The National R&D Programme on The Evaluation of Methods to Promote the Implementation of Research Findings*. Programme Report, NHS Executive, London, 2000.

17 Using evidence in practice: setting priorities in Oxfordshire

SIAN GRIFFITHS

> **Key messages**
> - Resources for healthcare are finite and difficult choices have to be made.
> - Evidence of clinical and cost effectiveness can help this decision making process if placed within an ethical framework, which also considers equity and patient choice.
> - The Priorities Forum engages all partners within the local healthcare system in the robust discussion of evidence, research findings and local implications of NICE guidance.
> - Newly emerging Primary Care Trusts wish to maintain the process despite the changing NHS structures.

Introduction

The NHS faces growing demands for health care as advances in treatment are made, new treatments become available, people live longer and are becoming more knowledgeable and articulate about treatment options. Resources continue to be limited, and the disparity between their availability and demand seems to be an eternal verity. In such a climate the health sector accepts that priority setting and rationing is necessary. Politicians find it more difficult to be explicit about the impossibility of meeting all the demands within existing resources and thus, access to some care needs to be restricted. So what are the criteria for such restrictions? And what role can evidence-based practice play?

Within Oxfordshire a process known as the Priorities Forum has developed with the aim of allowing decisions about difficult choices to be made within a framework of ethical values. It considers at a local level whether new drugs and treatments or treatments that are not routinely available should be funded, as well as discussing pressure points in local services and the impact of service developments. Using an ethical framework to support its decision making process, the Priorities Forum makes recommendations to the local health economy via the health authority board. In creating an environment where explicit, consistent and ethically sound decision making takes place, accountability to the public is possible.

This chapter describes the use of evidence within this decision making process.

The national approach in the UK

The need to be explicit about how resources were used was an integral part of the market culture of the 1990s – but explicit discussion of and the criteria for rationing was continuously avoided, despite the call in 1995 by a House of Commons Committee for a national debate to develop "an honest and realistic set of explicit, well understood ethical principles to guide the NHS into the next century".[1] In 1996, the King's Fund set up the Rationing Agenda Group[2] to widen the discussion, identifying the main questions:

- What range of services should be in the health care rationing debate?
- What is the range of ethically defensible criteria for deciding between competing claims and resources?
- Whose values should be taken into account?
- Who should undertake rationing?
- How will they be accountable?
- How explicit should rationing principles be?
- What information would be needed to make rationing more explicit and to hold decision makers more accountable?

These were bold questions at a time when inequalities in health were referred to as variations[3] and the limit to the funding available was not discussed openly. With the election of the Labour government in 1997, policy began to change. The internal market reforms were reversed and the New NHS[4] heralded a new focus on systemwide health care. A move to central policy making with local flexibility in implementation was apparent not only in the NHS Plan[5] but in the creation of central bodies essential to the overall notion of clinical governance. Clinical governance was to be delivered through improved clinical practice, better regulation, greater involvement of patients and new bodies such as the Commission for Health Improvement (CHI) and the National Centre for Clinical Effectiveness (NICE).

Locally this had implications for the role of evidence in decision making. The stimulus for the creation of the Priorities Forum had emerged in Oxfordshire because of the pressures on resources. The introduction of the culture of purchaser and provider had demanded greater clarity about what happened to the budget within Trusts. In general the currency used was numbers of cases or procedures and general guidelines were drawn up for what was and what was not included in the contract. Inevitably there were exceptions and this led to the introduction of extra contractual referrals (ECRs) for treatments which were not covered by routine contracts. Evidence was, at least in theory, one of the criteria used to set contracts – usually expressed in terms of quality.

ECRs produced pressures which highlighted the need for an additional system and criteria for decision making. Whilst as a tertiary specialist centre Oxford could have expected to be the recipient of contractual flows from other counties, there were certain groups of patients who needed to be referred out of county for care, notably those with mental health problems. In addition, because of the close relationships with the universities and their activities within research new ideas often emerged in advance of contract setting. The response was to create a forum for explicit decision making which included GPs, representatives from NHS Trusts and the public to consider requests for extra-contractual referrals.

Working through individual cases, case law was derived which was used to guide future decisions. General policy advice as well as individual requests for treatment were included on the agenda and results of discussions made widely known.

The terms of reference in Box 17.1 describe the workings of the Forum.

Box 17.1   Priorities Forum Terms of Reference

Oxfordshire Health Authority

Priorities Forum

Terms of Reference

1 Background
The Priorities Forum has existed in Oxfordshire since 1995. It was initially set up in the world of the internal market, and was particularly concerned with Extra Contractual Referrals (ECRs). Since 1997 and the change of government, it has continued to evolve in line with the modernisation agenda. At the present time the Primary Care Trusts (PCTs) have indicated they wish it to continue to provide advice, with particular reference to NICE guidance, specialist services, and new treatments which emerge from research.

Increasingly the Priorities Forum links with other counties. For example, the Public Health Resource Unit (PHRU) is co-ordinating a group to ensure common policies for expensive drugs in the Oxford Radcliffe Hospitals. The work continues to be supported by the Institute of Health Sciences, notably Professor Tony Hope on ethics and Alastair Gray and team on economics. A formal research project examining the economic values of relative decisions is also underway.

The key role of the Priorities Forum is to provide advice on prioritisation of issues considered by the health community. The recommendations and discussions of the Priorities Forum actively inform

---

continued

Box 17.1 *(continued)*

the Service and Financial Framework (SaFF) process and are linked to the Health Improvement Programme (HImP). Although not a decision making body, the Priorities Forum has an important role in steering health policy in Oxfordshire.

2 Current Status
The Priorities Forum is a sub-committee of the Health Authority. It has delegated powers to decide on individual patient cases presented to the Forum and to agree policy directions for issues considered. It reports formally to the Health Authority Board on recommendations made.

3 Terms of Reference
The Priorities Forum exists to provide an arena for policy discussions with a particular focus on priorities for health and health care within Oxfordshire. These discussions lead to explicit recommendations about what health care should be provided in the county, specifically in the following areas:

- New treatments (drugs, new indications for existing drugs, other procedures or therapeutic interventions)
- Treatments not routinely available
- Local implementation of recommendations from NICE – National Institute for Clinical Excellence, and guidance on other national priorities.

In making these recommendations the priorities forum will:

- Ensure decisions are made in accordance with the principles of its ethical framework (effectiveness, equity and patient choice)
- Engage in clinical discussions with Trusts
- Consider input from HA committees and groups, including APCO – Area Prescribing Committee, Oxfordshire
- Ensure appropriate links made with HImP groups
- Consider the health and service impact of priorities in key areas
- Ensure decisions are fed into SaFF negotiations.

4 Membership of the Forum
The chair of the forum will be the Director of Public Health.

The Forum members are drawn from:

Primary care   Representatives from primary care, including representatives from Primary Care Trusts and the Local Medical Committee of GPs.

Oxfordshire Health Authority   Executive and non-executive directors and selected specialists in commissioning and public health (the Chairperson and

Chief Executive of the Health Authority are not members of the Forum because they handle appeals against decisions).

continued

Box 17.1 *(continued)*

NHS Trusts   Medical directors and clinicians, including nurses and professions allied to medicine Senior Managers.

Institute of Health Sciences   Academic input includes Ethical and Health Economics support and medical students as part of the Public Health course.

Representatives of Oxfordshire Community Health Council   CHC representatives have the right to attend as observers. The CHC Chair and Secretary may speak at the Forum without compromising the CHC's role as public advocates.

Others on an ad hoc basis   The composition of the Forum shall be recorded in the Annual Report of the Authority.

5 Secretary
The Secretary of the Forum shall be the Clinical Effectiveness Co-ordinator from the Public Health Directorate.

6 Frequency of meetings
The Priorities Forum will meet on a monthly basis with the exception of June, when an annual seminar will be held to reflect on the work of the Priorities Forum over the previous year, and discuss areas for development. Ad hoc meetings of the Forum to discuss special issues may be convened when the chairperson deems it necessary.

7 Means of reporting
A formal agenda will be agreed for each meeting. Minutes of meetings and relevant papers will be sent to all members in advance. A report from the meeting will be presented to the next Health Authority board meeting. Monthly summary headlines are widely disseminated to the health community.

8 Appeals process
The appeals process is detailed in Priorities Forum policy statement no. 24 (1998) which forms an appendix to the terms of reference.

9 Disseminating decisions
Decisions are disseminated by lavender statements, reports to the HA and in monthly summary headlines to Primary Care

10 Quorum for decisions
As a sub-committee of the Health Authority, two members of the Health Authority (including associate members) need to be present for major financial decisions to be agreed.

11 Review
The Terms of Reference and membership of the Forum will be reviewed annually.

January 2001

Using evidence

The Priorities Forum acts as the focal point for complex decisions about new treatments which have resource implications – a sort of value for money test. Its decision making process is based on three key ethical values.[6] These are evidence of effectiveness – both clinical and cost; equity; patient choice. As a three legged stool, these values need to be traded off in the decision making process to maintain balance in our approach. The purpose of the Priorities Forum's ethical framework is threefold:

- It provides a coherent structure for discussion, ensuring all important aspects of each issue are considered
- It ensures consistency in decision making from meeting to meeting and with regard to different clinical topics
- It gives the forum a means of expressing the reasons behind the decisions made, particularly important for the appeals procedure.

Effectiveness

Effectiveness is the extent to which a health care intervention (a treatment, procedure or service) achieves an improvement for patients. The forum considers evidence of effectiveness from research findings whenever it makes a decision or recommendation. The evidence falls broadly into three categories:

- If there is good evidence that a treatment is ineffective then clearly it should not be funded
- If there is good evidence that an intervention is effective, then it may or may not be funded, depending on other criteria such as value in terms of relative benefit compared with other interventions
- In many cases, there is little firm evidence to conclude whether an intervention is effective or not. Interventions that fall into this category may or may not be funded. Here the Priorities Forum has to make a judgement about the likely effectiveness without good quality evidence.

Equity

Priorities Forum decisions are also formulated on the basis of equity, the core principle of which is that people in similar situations should be treated similarly. There should be no discrimination on the grounds of employment status, family circumstances, lifestyle, learning difficulty, age, race, sex, social position, financial status, religion or place of abode. Health-care should be allocated justly and fairly on the basis of need, and in terms of maximising the welfare of patients within the budget available. The forum tries to balance these approaches using a two step process, firstly considering the cost-effectiveness of the intervention for example using QALYs (Quality Adjusted Life Years); secondly if the intervention is less cost-effective than interventions normally funded, it considers whether there are, nevertheless reasons for funding it. Such reasons would include:

- **urgent need** for example life saving treatment
- **treatment for those whose quality of life is severely affected by chronic illness** for example patients with Multiple Sclerosis
- **justification for a treatment of high expense due to characteristic of the patient** for example the same level of dental care should be offered to people with learning disabilities as the rest of the population, even if it is less cost effective because more specialised services are needed.

Patient choice

Patient choice is considered by the forum to be important in reaching decisions about priorities for health care. The collective views of patient groups and those of individual patients are taken into account in the decision making process. The forum recognises that people need access to relevant information to help them make choices. The value of patient choice has three implications for the work of the forum:

- In assessing research on the effectiveness of interventions it is important to look at outcome measures which matter to patients
- Within those health care interventions that are purchased, patients should be enabled to make their own choices about which they want
- Each patient is unique. The forum recognises that some people may have a better chance than others of benefiting from a particular treatment.

However, patient choice is not the only criterion, and restricted resources mean that the Priorities Forum often has to refuse access to treatment. The authority will not make an exception simply because a patient chooses it, since this would deny another patient access to more effective treatment. The forum therefore has to carefully balance the components of its ethical framework.

Affordability

Each new development is considered initially within the framework of existing clinical practice – the envelope of resource.

The preparation for presentation of a case includes an independent search of the evidence for clinical effectiveness information. When a case

213

for supporting a clinical development is made, consideration should be given to:

- Whether a development can be funded by substituting a treatment of less value
- If demand is increasing, the criteria which are being used to agree the threshold of treatment
- If neither of the above is possible, which other service could receive a smaller resource.

Answering these questions relies on understanding relative impacts of a range of treatments and the quality of care they may provide. It also requires a clear understanding of the level at which intervention has been shown to be effective, as well as the level of care which is affordable. It is easier to answer the question of whether a treatment can be substituted with the same envelope of resource than it is to answer the question of whether a treatment for cardiac disease is of greater value than treatment for mental illness. It is also easier to make these decisions for drugs which have undergone trials and may effect a cure or at least diminution of symptoms whereas interventions which trade off over longer time periods or which improve quality of life rather than increasing survival are more difficult to consider. In such cases evidence may not exist. At such times the "common sense" test needs to be evoked. Lack of evidence should not preclude funding treatments as long as the reasons are understood and the regimen kept under review.

Communication

An essential element of the decision making process is communication of the decisions and the reasoning behind them. This is achieved through a variety of mechanisms.

Headlines

A document "Headlines from Priorities Forum" is produced as a monthly summary to communicate the key recommendations and issues from the forum in a short accessible format (two sides A4) for primary care. Headlines are widely disseminated to the health community, including distribution to all primary care practices.

Lavender statements

When policy is formulated, a policy document, known as a "lavender statement" is produced and disseminated widely to all primary care practices and across the health community.

Reporting to the Health Authority

A summary report from the forum is presented to the next public Health Authority board meeting.

Public leaflet

A Priorities Forum information leaflet is available for members of the public.

Web site

A Priorities Forum website is being developed which gives access to a background document on the forum, all lavender statements, the terms of reference, the public leaflet, latest "Headlines" and links and references to articles on priority setting.

Responding to change

The Priorities Forum has played a key role in ensuring open and fair decision making. However, its origins lie within a previous political environment in which there was more local autonomy and less explicit guidance on standards. The current political environment is much more directive about what standards can be expected and what care provided. This centralisation of policy is effected through a variety of bodies, but the one of most relevance to the Priorities Forum is NICE. Set up to undertake systematic appraisal of health interventions, NICE provides clinicians and managers with clear guidelines on what treatments work best for patients and which do not. The local impact is that technical appraisals and guidelines which are evidence-based are made widely available – thus reducing some of the work of the Forum. It is no longer necessary to undertake the appraisal – or expect to receive a variety of appraisals from different sources.

But NICE documents pose new challenges. The first is to assess current practice in the county and decide how well it measures up to the guidance and where there is room for improvement. For example, at a recent meeting of the forum the *Technology Appraisal Guidance: Guidance on the use of debriding agents and specialist wound care clinics for difficult to heal surgical wounds* and also *Clinical Guideline: Pressure ulcer risk assessment and prevention* were reviewed. The discussion which ensued identified that there were some problems in reaching the standards laid down because of lack of a coordinated approach and appropriate training for staff. This will require resources that will need to be found to address this gap.

In addition, NICE guidance is not simply accepted without discussion against the ethical criteria of the Forum. Shortage of resources is still a fact of life and NICE does not take into account issues of affordability. The health care economy, however, must consider affordability. With the flow of NICE documents becoming faster, the PF has a role in filtering and agreeing thresholds of interventions and envelopes of resources for each recommendation so that treatments are available locally. This may mean phasing in the introduction of a new drug over time to ensure the resources are made available.

At the same time as there is centralisation of guidance there is greater fragmentation of local decision making through the creation of Primary Care Trusts. A somewhat mixed message is given to PCTs, who are on the one hand told they are to have 75% of the NHS resources but on the other are told they need to follow national guidelines – not only through NICE but also through the National Service Frameworks and other central initiatives. Within Oxfordshire, with its five PCTs and county based structure for 600 000 population, there is general agreement that the Priorities Forum has an important part to play in co-ordinating NICE policies across the county, identifying where gaps may exist and where resources are particularly tight. Only time will tell whether this process will remain of value.

Looking to the future

The role of the Priorities Forum in implementing evidence-based care at a local level continues to develop. The Forum has moved away from deriving case law through individual patient dilemmas. Consideration of such issues as the need for cosmetic surgery or tattoo removal have been tested against the ethical framework and policy statements produced and disseminated. It now spends a greater proportion of its time bridging the gap between producing national guidance and ensuring its implementation – which has to occur within limited resources. It continues to review evidence produced by clinicians for new treatments and innovations and to recommend, or not, their development to all partners in the healthcare economy. It continues to try to communicate effectively with the public, recognizing that more needs to be done to engage them with the process and increase understanding of the dilemmas of making best use of limited resources.

Acknowledgement

I would like to thank Jane Harrison and Allison Thorpe for their help in preparing this chapter, and Tony Hope and John Reynolds for their contributions to the Forum.

216

References

1 House of Commons Hansard Debates, Volume 253, 31 January 1995.
2 New B. *The Rationing Agenda in the NHS*. London: King's Fund, 1996.
3 Health Service Guidelines. *Variations in Health*: Report of the Variations Sub-group of the Chief Medical Officer's Health of the Nation Working Group, HSG 54. London: Department of Health 1995.
4 Health Service Circular. *The New NHS: Modern, Dependable*. HSC 190. London: Department of Health 1998.
5 Secretary of State for Health. *The NHS Plan*. Command Paper, 4818-1. London: The Stationery Office, 2000.
6 Griffiths S, Reynolds J, Hope T. Priority Setting in Practice, in Coulter and Ham eds, *The Global Challenge of Health care Rationing*. Milton Keynes, The Open University, 2000.

Index

Page numbers in *italic* type refer to tables or boxed material; those in **bold** refer to figures

Printed in the United Kingdom
by Lightning Source UK Ltd.
127965UK00002B/115-117/A